Hormone Replacement Therapy and the Menopause

Edited by

Michael S Marsh MD MRCOG
*Consultant & Senior Lecturer in Obstetrics
and Gynaecology
Department of Obstetrics & Gynaecology
King's College Hospital, London, UK*

Juliet E Compston MD FRCPath FRCP FMedSci
*Reader in Metabolic Bone Disease &
Honorary Consultant Physician
University of Cambridge School of Clinical
Medicine, Cambridge, UK*

MARTIN DUNITZ

© 2002 Martin Dunitz Ltd, a member of the Taylor & Francis group

First published in the United Kingdom in 2002
by Martin Dunitz Ltd, The Livery House, 7–9 Pratt Street, London NW1 0AE

Tel: +44 (0) 20 7482 2202
Fax: +44 (0) 20 7267 0159
E-mail: info@dunitz.co.uk
Website: http://www.dunitz.co.uk

Although every effort has been made to ensure that all owners of copyright material have been
acknowledged in this publication, we would be glad to acknowledge in subsequent reprints or editions
any omissions brought to our attention.

A CIP for this book is available from the British Library.

ISBN 1-85317-691-5

A 030009

Distributed in the USA by
Fulfilment Center
Taylor & Francis
7625 Empire Drive
Florence, KY 41042, USA
Toll Free Tel.: +1 800 634 7064
E-mail: cserve@routledge_ny.com

Distributed in Canada by
Taylor & Francis
74 Rolark Drive
Scarborough, Ontario M1R 4G2, Canada
Toll Free Tel.: +1 877 226 2237
E-mail: tal_fran@istar.ca

WP 580

Distributed in the rest of the world by
ITPS Limited
Cheriton House
North Way
Andover, Hampshire SP10 5BE, UK
Tel.: +44 (0)1264 332424
E-mail: reception@itps.co.uk

Composition by Wearset Ltd, Boldon, Tyne and Wear
Printed and bound in Great Britain by The Cromwell Press, Trowbridge.

Contents

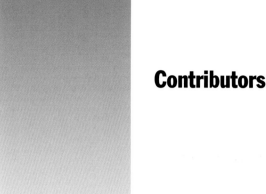

Contributors

Linda Cardozo MD FRCOG
Professor of Urogynaecology, King's College Hospital, Denmark Hill, London SE5 9RS, UK

Juliet E Compston MD FRCPath FRCP FMedSci
Reader in Metabolic Bone Disease and Honorary Consultant Physician, University of Cambridge School of Clinical Medicine, Addenbrooke's Hospital, Hills Road, Cambridge CB2 2QQ, UK

Alison Cooper MB BS MRCOG
Senior Registrar, Department of Obstetrics & Gynaecology, King's College Hospital, Denmark Hill, London SE5 9RS, UK

David Crook PhD
Senior Research Fellow, Department of Cardiovascular Biochemistry, St Bartholomew's and The Royal London School of Medicine, Charterhouse Square, London EC1M 6BQ, UK

Andrew Hextall MRCOG
Specialist Registrar in Urogynaecology, Department of Urogynaecology, King's College Hospital, Denmark Hill, London SE5 9RS, UK

Myra Hunter PhD CPsychol AFBPS
Head, Department of Clinical Health
Psychology/Senior Lecturer, St Thomas'
Hospital, Lambeth Palace Road,
London SE1 7EH, UK

Clare E Kearney MB ChB MRCOG
Research Fellow, Centre for Metabolic Bone
Disease, University of Hull, Hull Royal
Infirmary, H S Brocklehurst Building,
220–236 Anlaby Road, Hull HU3 2RW, UK

Jo Marsden BSc FRCS
Specialist Registrar in General Surgery, The
Royal Surrey County Hospital, Egerton Road,
Guildford, Surrey GU2 5XX, UK

Michael S Marsh MD MRCOG
Consultant and Senior Lecturer in Obstetrics
and Gynaecology, Department of Obstetrics
& Gynaecology, King's College Hospital,
Denmark Hill, London SE5 9RS, UK

Declan Murphy MD MRCPsych
Professor in Brain Maturation and Psychiatry,
and Honorary Consultant Psychiatrist,
Department of Psychological Medicine,
Institute of Psychiatry, De Crespigny Park,
London SE5 8AF, UK

Bent Ottesen MD DrMedSci
Professor, Department of Obstetrics &
Gynaecology, Hvidovre Hospital, University
of Copenhagen, Copenhagen, Denmark

David W Purdie MD, FRCOG, FRCP(Ed)
Head of Clinical Research, Centre for
Metabolic Bone Disease, University of Hull,
Hull Royal Infirmary, H S Brocklehurst
Building, 220–236 Anlaby Road,
Hull HU3 2RW, UK

Régine Sitruk-Ware MD
Adjunct Professor, Rockfeller University, and
Executive Director, Contraceptive
Development, Center for Biomedical
Research, 1230 York Avenue, New York,
NY 10021, USA

John C Stevenson MB BS FRCP FESC
Reader and Honorary Consultant,
Endocrinology and Metabolic Medicine,
Imperial College School of Medicine, Mint
Wing, St Mary's Hospital, Praed Street,
London W2 1NY, UK

Anette Tønnes Pedersen MD PhD
Consultant, Department of Obstetrics
& Gynaecology, Hvidovre
Hospital, University of Copenhagen,
Copenhagen, Denmark

Therese van Amelsvoort MD MSc MRCPsych
Specialist Registrar in Psychiatry and Clinical
Research Worker, Department
of Psychological Medicine, Institute
of Psychiatry, De Crespigny Park,
London SE5 8AF, UK

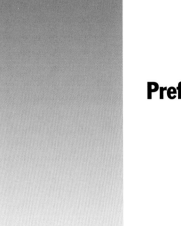

Preface

The number of women living to retirement and beyond is likely to continue to grow in future years. An increasingly well-informed postmenopausal population is likely to seek the advice of their physician or specialist nurse about the risks and benefits of HRT and other therapies for the prevention of conditions related to oestrogen deficiency, such as osteoporosis, cardiovascular disease and Alzheimer's disease. *Hormone Replacement Therapy and the Menopause* aims to provide the clinician with information that can be passed on to women so that they may make informed choices about their care. Information is also included that will help the practising clinician manage women taking HRT, both those who are having difficulties with treatment, and those who are not.

Many of the principles of managing and counselling women taking HRT have changed considerably over the last five years in the light of fresh research, and these shifts are especially reflected in the chapters dealing with cardiovascular disease, lipids and lipoproteins, vascular flow, osteoporosis, the breast and Alzheimer's disease.

'Designer' oestrogens in the form of selective oestrogen receptor modulators (SERMs) are given their own chapter.

More SERMs are likely to be developed and may in the long term provide a method of treatment that incorporates all of the advantages and none of the disadvantages of conventional HRT.

Although appropriate counselling of women seeking HRT becomes more difficult as old 'certainties' become uncertainties, we hope that this book will aid the clinician and nurse in giving evidence-based advice to their patients.

Michael S Marsh
Juliet E Compston

Monitoring and management

Alison Cooper, Michael S Marsh

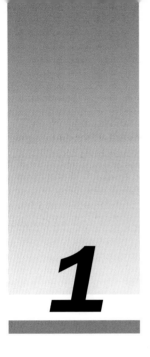

Introduction

Demographic changes over the next 20 years will mean that
the number of people living to retirement and beyond will
increase substantially. If we are to help protect women from
the problems of oestrogen deficiency, such as osteoporosis,
cardiovascular disease and possibly Alzheimer's disease, we
must provide easy access to health care advice, together with
unbiased information upon which the patient can make an
informed decision about whether or not to take hormone
replacement therapy (HRT). We must also make adequate
provision for managing and monitoring these patients once
HRT is started.

Assessment and monitoring

Many women seeking medical advice about problems arising
from oestrogen deficiency may not have had contact with a
doctor for many years. It would therefore seem wise to use
this contact not only to discuss menopausal issues, but to
screen for problems relating to personal and family factors.

The initial consultation should include a medical and

gynaecological history, as well as a personal or family history of arterial and thromboembolic disease, breast, ovarian and colon cancer, diabetes, osteoporosis or liver disease.

A general physical examination, including height, weight and blood pressure, should be performed. The breasts should be examined and a pelvic examination undertaken.

If risk factors have been identified, it may then be necessary to perform other investigations.

- A patient with a personal, first- or second-degree family history of venous thromboembolic disease should have a thrombophilia and coagulation screen performed, e.g. kaolin cephalin clotting time (KCCT), antithrombin III, protein C and S and activated protein C resistance (factor V Leiden mutation).
- A fasting lipid profile should be performed in women with a relevant family history of early-onset arterial disease.
- A patient with a relevant family history of breast cancer should be considered for screening mammography, whether or not HRT is taken.
- Occasionally, serum follicle-stimulating hormone (FSH) and luteinizing hormone (LH) may be useful, for example in confirming premature menopause. However, in the perimenopausal woman FSH and LH

values may change every 2 hours and are of little predictive value.
- Bone density measurements may be appropriate in women with risk factors who do not wish to take HRT unless low bone density is proven to be low.

Presenting accurate information about the benefits and risks of HRT in an impartial manner will enable most women to make an informed decision regarding treatment.

Before a patient starts HRT it is important that potential side-effects are discussed. These include leg cramps, nausea and breast tenderness, which usually resolve spontaneously within the first few weeks.[1] Patients should be asked to monitor the pattern of withdrawal bleeding. The need for regular surveillance should be explained. The first follow-up visit is usually after 3 months. Patients should also be given details of whom to contact should they need advice. Compliance is likely to be better if women feel confident with their therapy and know who to contact if they experience problems.

Monitoring

At the first visit after starting HRT, the patient should be asked whether symptoms are controlled and whether side-effects have occurred. The maximum benefits in relieving flushes and sweats are not achieved until the third month of therapy. Continued nipple sensitivity and leg cramps suggest that consideration should be given to reducing the dose of oestrogen.

It is important in women taking sequential combined therapy to find out whether withdrawal bleeding has occurred and, if so, its timing, amount and duration. Women on continuous combined therapy may still be experiencing some light bleeding, but this should be resolving by three months.

The patient's weight and blood pressure are traditionally measured at each visit. Weight gain is a common complaint at the menopause and body weight increases on average 1 kg a year around this time,[2] but many placebo-controlled studies have demonstrated that HRT does not increase weight. Some women on HRT may experience symptoms such as bloating and fluid retention, which can often be helped by altering either the dose, the route or the type of administration of HRT. Women should be encouraged to adopt a healthy lifestyle, paying regard to diet and exercise.

There is no evidence that HRT increases blood pressure. However, there are occasional reports of idiosyncratic rises in blood pressure. These are difficult to explain and may not be related to HRT, because for the most part the oestrogens in HRT preparations are structurally identical to those produced by the ovary, and most preparations deliver much less than did the ovary during the reproductive years.

Further visits usually occur at 12–18-month intervals, or earlier if a problem arises.

Management
Side-effects of HRT
Vaginal bleeding

In women who have an intact uterus it is important to administer a progesterone in order to protect the endometrium against hyperplasia and neoplasia.[3] Progestogens should be administered for at least 12 days in each 28-day treatment cycle. The types and dosages of oral progestogens in current use are listed in *Table 1.1*.

Roughly 85% of women receiving sequential HRT will have a withdrawal bleed, which occurs either at the end of or immediately after the progesterone phase of treatment. Occasionally women do not bleed. This is more common in those who are many years beyond the menopause.

Once a woman has been amenorrhoeic for at least 12 months, she can convert to a 'no-bleed' continuous combined HRT in which progestogens are given daily in combination with an oestrogen, rendering the endometrium atrophic.

Abnormal bleeding is defined as heavy and/or prolonged bleeding at the appropriate time in the cycle, or breakthrough bleeding which occurs at any other time. In women taking continuous combined HRT there

Table 1.1
Recommended daily dose of progesterone needed for endometrial protection when prescribed as part of sequential HRT

C19 androgenic progesterones	
Levonorgestrel	150 mg
Norethisterone acetate	0.7–1.0 mg
C21 less androgenic progesterones	
Medroxyprogesterone acetate	10 mg
Dydrogesterone	10–20 mg
Progesterone	200–400 mg

should be no bleeding. However, approximately 40% of postmenopausal women commencing continuous combined HRT will experience bleeding during the first 3–6 months. One study suggested that only 40–50% of women still bleeding after 6–8 months of treatment eventually achieved amenorrhoea after a further 12 months.[4]

There are no accepted criteria for the management of abnormal bleeding with continuous combined therapy, but it would seem prudent to investigate women who continue to or start to bleed after the first 6 months.

Causes of abnormal bleeding

Constitutional

Women who experience prolonged heavy bleeding during their reproductive years are more likely to experience this pattern with HRT use. Reducing the oestrogen dose may help, but this may compromise symptom control and may reduce the beneficial effects on the cardiovascular and skeletal systems.

Failure of compliance

This is probably the most common cause of breakthrough bleeding. Missing one or two tablets, or forgetting to change a patch at the correct time, can lead to breakthrough bleeding. Women who find the progestogenic side-effects of HRT intolerable often omit the progestogen. If progesterone is often omitted, bleeding often becomes chaotic and endometrial hyperplasia and carcinoma may develop.

Previous oestrogen implant therapy

Oestradiol implants can continue to release oestradiol for up to 3 years following insertion.[5] Patients should therefore be advised to continue using progestogens for 12 days each calendar month until there has been no withdrawal bleeding for 3 consecutive months.

Drug interactions

Enzyme inducers such as phenytoin, carbamazepine, rifampicin and barbiturates increase the activity of liver enzymes responsible for liver metabolism and coaccelerate oestrogen clearance. Antibiotics can cause intestinal 'hurry' and alter bowel flora, thereby increasing the chances of breakthrough bleeding. St John's wort also interacts with oestrogens.

Stress, especially if it includes long-distance travel

The mechanism of action is unknown, but may involve poor compliance.

Poor gastrointestinal absorption

Bowel disorders such as Crohn's disease, ulcerative colitis and Whipple's disease may all affect the absorption of oestrogens and progestogens from the gut. In practice it is probably advisable for these women to have transdermal or subcutaneous therapy.

Failure to synchronize endogenous ovarian activity with exogenous hormone treatment

In pre- or perimenopausal women who still have a regular 28-day cycle it is important to administer the progestogen starting on the 17th day of the cycle, so as to coincide with endogenous production of progesterone. Failure to do so will result in patients bleeding twice during the cycle, once because of their own ovarian function and once because of HRT.

HRT and tamoxifen use

Tamoxifen is associated with an increased risk of developing endometrial polyps and endometrial carcinoma.[6] In women who combine HRT and tamoxifen and experience abnormal vaginal bleeding, hysteroscopy and endometrial biopsy is advised. Ultrasound assessment of the endometrium in women on tamoxifen shows thickening of the endometrium with cystic spaces. There is currently no established correlation between endometrial histology and ultrasound findings.

Gynaecological disorders
Fibroids

Fibroids are oestrogen dependent and can enlarge significantly with HRT. If this occurs in a woman who wishes to remain on HRT then surgical intervention is usually required; this involves either hysterectomy, or myomectomy, either via laparatomy or minimally invasive procedures.

Endometrial polyps

These can cause heavy withdrawal bleeding, breakthrough bleeding or bloody vaginal discharge. They can often be detected by transvaginal ultrasound and can be removed by hysteroscopic resection.

Endometrial hyperplasia and carcinoma

These are best diagnosed by endometrial sampling. Women who develop endometrial cancer while on HRT appear to have a better prognosis than those who have not taken HRT.[7]

Adenomyosis

This is more common in women in their fourth and fifth decades, often presenting with menorrhagia, dyspareunia and dysmenorrhoea. It is most commonly diagnosed after endometrial resection or hysterectomy, but can sometimes be diagnosed preoperatively by transvaginal ultrasound or nuclear magnetic resonance imaging.

Ovarian tumours, cervical carcinoma, and vaginal or vulval lesions are all causes of abnormal bleeding. The investigation and management of these are not within the scope of this book.

Management and investigation of abnormal bleeding

It is important to take a careful history to exclude obvious reasons for abnormal bleeding. Women taking sequential therapy, or those who experience bleeding too early in the progesterone phase of treatment, may benefit from increasing the dose of progestogen. The persistence of heavy, prolonged or erratic bleeding demands investigation.

Transvaginal ultrasound

This can be used to assess endometrial thickness in postmenopausal women on continuous combined therapy. Where the endometrium is more than 4 mm thick an endometrial biopsy and/or hysteroscopy should be undertaken. Ultrasound may also detect the presence of polyps, fibroids, endometriosis and adenomyosis.

Outpatient endometrial biopsy

The most commonly used devices for outpatient endometrial sampling are the

Pipelle and the Vabra curettes. Pipelle curettage samples less of the endometrial surface than does the Vabra – 4% and 42%, respectively[8] – but the Vabra causes greater discomfort. It is best to sample the endometrium in the oestrogenic/progestogenic phase of the cycle as sampling at this phase allows the degree of secretory change to be assessed and it is easier to differentiate between secretory and hyperplastic endometrium than between proliferative and hyperplastic endometrium. The disadvantage of these methods is that they are a 'blind' procedure and endometrial polyps may be missed. If abnormal bleeding persists then hysteroscopic assessment should be undertaken.

Hysteroscopy

This can be performed under local or general anaesthesia. The whole of the endometrium can be visualized, and polyps, submucous fibroids and abnormal endometrium can be biopsied.

Progestogenic and oestrogenic intolerance

Most problems with HRT arise from the progestogen, which can cause any or all of the symptoms outlined in *Table 1.2*. If symptoms arise, the dose and duration of progestogen can be reduced. However, the patient must be made aware that doing so may increase the risk of endometrial carcinoma.

If progestogenic side-effects occur, it is often worth substituting an androgenic progestogen for a less androgenic one, as the latter probably cause fewer side-effects. An approved natural progesterone (e.g. Cyclogest (Shire Pharmaceuticals Ltd, Basingstoke, UK) or Crinone (Serono Pharmaceuticals Ltd, Feltham, UK), may also be tried.

Long-cycle therapy can be considered. In this regimen progestogen is added only every third month. However, the safety of this type of therapy concerning endometrial carcinoma is unclear and this should be made clear to patients considering this form of treatment.

The Mirena intrauterine system (Schering Health Care, Burgess Hill, UK) may be used. This treatment reduces menstrual blood flow and also acts as a contraceptive.

In a small proportion of women hysterectomy may be the only alternative if women with severe progestogenic side-effects wish to continue with HRT.

Table 1.2

Breast tenderness
Acne
Mood change/depression
Lower abdominal pain
Backache
Fluid retention

Table 1.3

General
Breast tenderness, nipple sensitivity
Nausea
Leg cramps
Headaches
Dyspepsia
Fluid retenion/bloating
Device-specific
Skin irritation
Poor adhesion
Local sepsis/scars from implants
Tachyphalaxis

As with progestogens, where there are oestrogenic side-effects (*Table 1.3*) reducing the dose of therapy or changing to an alternative route of delivery may be appropriate. Again, care must be taken when reducing the dose of oestrogen that symptoms are controlled and that adequate bone and cardiovascular protection is achieved.

There may be side-effects relating to the route of administration of therapy. Dyspepsia appears to occur in 3–4 % of women taking oral oestrogens. This can sometimes be abolished by taking the tablet at night, or with food. If this is unsuccessful a non-oral route can be considered. Skin irritation and poor adhesion can occur with patch therapy. If so, alternative patches may be tried or another route of administration used.

Where implants are used, occasionally the site of administration may become infected. An important potential problem with the use of implant therapy is tachyphylaxis. This is a phenomenon whereby insertion of the first implant is followed by a rapid rise in oestradiol levels and a plateau is reached after some weeks. As the oestradiol levels fall below this plateau the patient begins to experience a recurrence of symptoms, even though the plasma level of oestradiol is well within the normal premenopausal range. As the patient is symptomatic the practitioner inserts a further implant and there is a further rise in oestradiol levels. However, this rise is not maintained, and as the plasma level falls the patient once again becomes symptomatic. If this cycle is repeated then supraphysiological levels of oestradiol may develop. Some of these patients experience symptoms of oestrogen overdosage, such as nausea and breast tenderness.

The management of these patients is very difficult. The patient needs to go through a withdrawal period where the oestradiol falls to premenopausal levels, which may take 2 years. This often distressing experience can sometimes be helped by supplementing oestradiol in the form of patches or tablets. In women using implants plasma oestradiol levels should be checked regularly. It is probably best to avoid the insertion of further implants if the plasma oestradiol is greater than 600 pmol/l.

Management of women with endometriosis

Probably, the most important clinical problem in managing women with endometriosis is the use of HRT in women following total abdominal hysterectomy and bilateral salpingo-oöphorectomy for extensive disease, often involving the bowel or bladder. This history is not a contraindication to HRT, as ectopically sited endometrium may not behave in the same way as endometrium sited within the uterine cavity. It is wise to start with the lowest oestrogen dose that will control symptoms. It is unknown whether the addition of a progestogen protects against recurrence of the disease. It may be necessary to add testosterone to the oestrogen. It is important to advise the patient to report any symptoms or signs of disease recurrence, such as dyspareunia or pelvic pain.

Management of women with benign breast disease

Benign breast disease is not a contraindication to HRT. Certain forms of benign breast disease are known to increase the risk of breast cancer whether HRT is taken or not. These include lobular and ductal hyperplasia with atypia. Whether HRT increases the risk of breast cancer in women with these histological diagnoses is unknown.

Testosterone implants

Testosterone is an androgen produced by the ovary. Oöphorectomy removes this source. The physiological role of testosterone in women is unclear; however, following oöphorectomy some women experience loss of libido and a reduction in energy despite adequate oestradiol levels. These symptoms are often helped by the administration of testosterone implants. The dose most commonly used is 50–100 mg every 6–8 months. A potential side-effect is virilization, which includes hirsutism and deepening of the voice, but this is very rarely seen especially when low dose-therapy is used.

In the near future other routes of testosterone administration may become available, such as transdermal patches.

Duration of HRT therapy

The length of time women remain on treatment depends on the indication.

Vasomotor symptoms may last from 6 months to over 20 years.

In terms of fracture prevention, it appears that the effects of oestrogen therapy on the skeleton last for as long as treatment continues. Once treatment stops the beneficial effects start to be lost.

With regard to the prevention of cardiovascular disease, the beneficial effects appear to last while treatment is maintained, but again are lost when treatment stops. It is uncertain whether combined oestrogen and progestogen HRT produces the same effects on cardiovascular disease risk as oestrogen alone.

The major concern with long-term treatment is the risk of breast cancer. A recent large meta-analysis[9] of the women from 51 epidemiological studies reported that among current users of HRT, or those that had ceased use 1–4 years previously, the relative risk of having breast cancer diagnosed increased by a factor of 1.023 for each year of use. In this same group the relative risk was 1.35 with 5 years' use or longer. There was found to be an increase in risk of breast cancer in non-users of HRT who had a late menopause. In this group the relative risk was 1.028 for each year of ovarian function. Thus each year of exposure to HRT increased the risk of breast cancer by 2.3%. Each year of exposure to normal ovarian function with late menopause increased the risk of breast cancer by 2.8%. The analysis also reported that breast cancers diagnosed in women on HRT appeared to be localized to the breast. Whether the use of HRT produces less aggressive disease, or whether the cancers are detected earlier as a result of more vigilant surveillance, is unknown. Most studies agree that there is no increase risk in breast cancer in women who take HRT for less than 5 years.

Conclusion

Choosing the correct treatment from an ever-increasing array of new HRT products can appear daunting. However, once individual patient factors have been considered, such as the presence or absence of a uterus, peri- or postmenopausal state and the preferred route of administration, the choice is usually fairly straightforward. The final choice will be based on clinical experience and cost.

It is important that appropriate follow-up is arranged to resolve any side-effects or anxieties, and that patients know where to return to should they experience problems before their next appointment.

References

1.   Campbell S, Whitehead M. Oestrogen therapy and the menopausal syndrome. *Clin Obstet Gynecol* 1997; **4**: 31–47.

2.   Wing R, Matthews K, Kuller L *et al.* Weight gain at the time of menopause. *Arch Intern Med* 1991; **151**: 97–102.

3.   Whitehead M, Townsend P, Pryse-Davies J *et al.* Effects of estrogens and progestins on the biochemistry of the postmenopausal endometrium. *N Engl J Med* 1981; **305**: 1599–1605.

4.   Archer D, Pickar J, Bottiglioni F. Bleeding patterns in postmenopausal women taking continuous combined or sequential regimens of conjugated estrogens with medroxyprogesterone acetate. *Obstet Gynecol* 1994; **83**: 686–692.

5. Ganger K, Cust M, Whitehead M. Symptoms of oestrogen deficiency associated with supraphysiological plasma oestradiol concentrations in women with oestradiol implants. *Br Med J* 1989; **299**: 601–602.

6. Ismail S. Pathology of endometrium with tamoxifen. *J Clin Pathol* 1994; **47:** 827–833.

7. Nyholm H, Neilson A, Norup P. Endometrial cancer in postmenopausal women with and without previous estrogen replacement treatment : comparison of clinical and histopathological characteristics. *Gynecol Oncol* 1993; **49**: 229–235.

8. Rodriguez G, Yaqub N, King M. A comparison of the Pipelle device and the Vabra aspirator as measured by endometrial denudation in hysterectomy specimens: the Pipelle device samples significantly less of the endometrial surface than the Vabra aspirator. *Am J Obstet Gynecol* 1993; **168**: 55–59.

9. The Collaborative Group on Hormonal Factors in Breast Cancer. Hormone replacement therapy and breast cancer. *Lancet* 1997; **350**: 1047–1059.

Edition as

Psychological aspects of the menopause and hormone replacement therapy

Myra Hunter

2

Introduction

The nature of research into psychological aspects of the menopause and its treatment reflects the sociocultural meanings of menopause prevalent at the time. Gynaecological, psychiatric, and psychoanalytic writings of the early 20th century explored the experience of menopause by studying individual cases of women seeking help for particular problems. A negative view evolved and theories developed of menopause as a time of loss of femininity and sexuality to be mourned,[1] a potential form of psychosis,[2] and a type of 'hysteria' warranting gynaecological surgery.[3] Advances in biomedical research have led to the application of hormonal preparations to treat vasomotor symptoms, and as preventative strategies for osteoporosis and cardiovascular disease. More recently the potential effects of hormone replacement therapy (HRT) upon cognitive function and Alzheimer's disease, and upon quality of life in general have become growing areas of research. In parallel with biomedical research, psychological studies have focused upon measuring outcome and change in symptoms experienced during the menopause, as well as broader quality of life measures.

Since the 1970s social scientists have questioned the assumption that the menopause is a 'deficiency disease' and, by carrying out general population, prospective studies, have provided data that point to a less pathological view of the menopause. There is no conclusive evidence that clinical depression increases during the menopause.[4] Studies of psychological symptoms generally show few changes across stages of the menopause.[5–7] Furthermore, when well-being was measured in a cross-sectional and prospective Australian study of the menopause transition, no effects of menopausal status were found.[8] Despite the fact that a wide variety of physical and psychological symptoms have been attributed to hormone changes during the menopause— such as irritability, headaches, depression, anxiety, weight gain, aches and pains, poor memory and concentration, and loss of libido—hot flushes and night sweats (vasomotor symptoms) are the only definite symptoms of the menopause.[9] Even if symptoms are reported by women in surveys this does not necessarily mean that the symptoms are problematic. Porter and colleagues[10] asked a random sample of 6084 Scottish women whether they experienced a number of symptoms and then whether they perceived them to be a problem. Vasomotor symptoms and atrophic vaginal changes were the only symptoms to be associated with menopausal status; 57% reported having hot flushes and 22% regarded these as a problem.

Other general somatic and psychological symptoms were reported but were perceived as problematic by approximately 10% and 20%, respectively. For example, 51% and 58% experienced depression and anxiety, respectively, but only 22% and 26%, respectively described these experiences as a problem.

The use of more sophisticated methodologies has enabled researchers to examine factors that predict depressed mood and psychological distress during the menopause. Women who are depressed before the menopause and those who experience psychosocial problems at the time, such as life stress, bereavement, economic and family problems, are more likely to report depression during the menopause.[7,11] In addition, negative beliefs about the menopause held before the menopause are associated with reports of psychological symptoms during the menopause.[11] The experience of prolonged vasomotor symptoms during the perimenopause is associated with psychological distress, and research suggests that particular health problems—chronic arthritis and thyroid problems—increase the risk of chronic depression during the menopause transition.[6] It is important to place this literature within the broader framework of studies of gender differences in psychological health. For example, Bebbington[12] reports that whereas the gender difference in psychological morbidity is 2:1 in favour of men during the reproductive years (20–55), this reduces markedly around the age of 55, after which age women report fewer psychological problems. In a recent study of 50-year-old men and women, we found that there were no significant gender differences in reports of life satisfaction and health-related quality of life.[13] Research carried out in different cultures also points to variation in the sociocultural factors that influence the personal and social significance of menopause and ageing. Anthropological studies provide examples of how menopause can be a positive event, particularly when it signifies a change in social status.[14] In general, women living in non-Western societies appear to report fewer symptoms at the menopause than those living in the West. However, it is likely that material differences, such as dietary and reproductive practices and levels of exercise, contribute to cross-cultural differences, as well as cultural values and the social position of middle-aged and older women.

In general this strand of research has focused on menopause as a normal developmental life stage and has provided evidence of the strong influence of psychosocial factors upon women's well-being. Another result of this research has been the development of standardized questionnaires to measure changes across the menopause transition, such as the Greene Climacteric Scale[15] and the Women's Health Questionnaire,[16] which have been

recommended to replace earlier scales, such as the Kupperman Index.[17] At the same time, studies of menopause clinic attenders, those seeking medical help for menopausal problems, have demonstrated consistently high levels of psychological distress, as well as vasomotor symptoms, in these populations.[18,19] In a study carried out in a London hospital, we found that seeking help from a menopause clinic was best predicted by reports of psychological symptoms together with vasomotor symptoms in the context of certain beliefs—that the menopause was a disease-like process.[20] These findings and reports from clinicians have resulted in debates about how best to treat psychological symptoms in these samples of women. Current treatments include HRT, antidepressants, and psychological treatment (cognitive behaviour therapy). Further research is needed to clarify the relative effectiveness of these treatments and also the treatment preferences of middle-aged women with clinical depression who are seeking help.

In the sections that follow, three areas of research are presented that illustrate the kinds of research questions, theories, and methodologies that are currently being considered in psychological research on the menopause and HRT. These include (1) qualitative studies of experience of the menopause, (2) studies of decision making in relation to hormonal treatments, and (3) psychological interventions for middle-aged women.

Qualitative studies of experience of the menopause

Given the different theoretical perspectives that frame the meaning of the menopause, ranging from deficiency disease to normal developmental phase, it is often difficult to now how closely these models match women's own experience or the extent to which women draw upon different theoretical models when describing their own menopause. From a woman's perspective the menopause has acquired complex social and cultural meanings, being inextricably linked to age and often coinciding with life changes. For example, 'the change of life' in popular discourse reflects the view that the menopause might be paralleled by role changes and emotional and social adaptations that may occur during midlife. Concepts such as 'empty nest', physical decline, loss of femininity, loss of sexuality, involutional melancholia and vaginal atrophy have contributed to varied, but generally negative, stereotypes of menopausal women in Western cultures. When visiting a doctor a woman is likely to share her doctor's language and present symptoms and side-effects. What is not clear is how women themselves think about and discuss menopause—in other words what discourses they use—in other settings. In order to explore women's views and experiences of the menopause, we carried out a qualitative study of women's accounts of the menopause.[21]

Forty-five women aged 49–51 were recruited from the age/sex register of a general practice in North London, serving a large socially mixed area. Thirty-seven who were perimenopausal, postmenopausal, or taking HRT were asked about their lives, general health, and the menopause. The interviews were taped, transcribed, critically read by both investigators, and taken to a peer group discussion. Thematic discourse analysis was used to explore women's accounts of the impact of menopause.[22] Six broad themes were identified from the women's accounts, which are outlined briefly below.

Bodily changes

How women defined themselves in relation to the menopause tended to elicit discussion of physical changes, particularly hot flushes and night sweats. Menstrual and minor physical and emotional changes were mentioned but to a lesser extent. Descriptions of hot flushes and night sweats varied considerably between women, many viewing them as not problematic. For example:

Maybe, about two years ago I was feeling hot at times, hot flushes but no more. It wasn't for long. I get hot at times but it doesn't bother me. If it's hot I just open the window but otherwise I don't have any ill effects at all.

However, several found them troublesome and embarrassing and there was a general concern about other people's reactions:

> *The first time I got it I felt that everyone was looking at me; I used to go bright red and feel embarrassed. It only lasted a few minutes but does happen sometimes when I'm talking to people now: I feel uncomfortable. All the blood rushes to my face.*

Hot flushes were experienced as more problematic in certain situations, for example in situations in which they could not easily take steps to cool down, and when disrupted sleep affected ability to deal with work. Therefore the experience of hot flushes and night sweats was variable and partly influenced by the woman's social context and lifestyle.

Menopause as non-event: continuation of the self

The most commonly voiced theme was that the menopause had no or few consequences for the women at all. They tended to describe themselves as not particularly changed by the menopause:

> *It hasn't made me anything better or anything worse. I feel no different in myself.*

Accounts of bodily changes were to some extent separated from how they felt the menopause had impacted upon themselves:

> *I didn't like my periods being irregular or my body feeling different but in myself, well, I still felt that inside I hadn't changed.*

No more periods

Cessation of menstruation was seen as a positive change by all the women who commented on menstrual changes. Menstruation was generally talked about as something negative and relief was expressed about its absence:

> *It's nice to get it over with and not have periods any more.*

Relief was expressed particularly by women who had had heavy or problematic menstrual periods.

Menopause as change in reproductive stage

Although there was a general awareness that the menopause marked the end of a woman's reproductive phase of life, the majority did not express unhappiness about this. Reproductive decisions tended to have been made earlier in their lives.

> *I never really wanted to have children so it never really worried me in that way. I'll be quite pleased in some ways.*

It won't make any difference for me because I was sterilized at 38 and I won't feel that I can't have children any more because I've been quite happy not having children for the last 12 years.

Women's accounts challenged the view of the menopausal woman mourning the loss of fertility, although particular circumstances (such as the earlier death of a child) influenced the individual meaning of the menopause as a reproductive event.

Menopause as a sign of ageing

The menopause was inextricably associated with age. Being 50 and menopause were used interchangeably. Although the majority challenged the view that menopause necessarily marks the beginning of old age, some women did voice concerns about ageing and fears about being old:

I think once the menopause is over you feel as though you're fast approaching retirement and it doesn't seem so very long now to being old. It's a bit frightening that it's only a few years away and there's still lots of things to do. I think in ten years time I'll be old.

However, a more positive perspective relating to age, voiced by several women, was of the menopause as a time for reflection:

It brings home to you that perhaps you're in

the last half of life . . . It's a time for a bit of reflection about where you're going over the next few years.

Social context was again an important influence on perceptions of ageing. One woman who worked with teenagers in an office had become increasingly aware of feeling different from them and aware of her age:

I've never looked at myself as being in my 50s but I find that I do feel it more now ... because I'm working with people that are 17, 18, and I feel older now. It suddenly makes you think God I'm 50, where has my life gone, but before I never had these feelings at all. I don't know whether it's to do with the menopause or not or just your working environment.

Staving off the unknown: menopause as unspoken taboo

Although the interviewer used the word 'menopause', the women tended not to. 'It' and 'this' were used, suggesting that the menopause was not commonly discussed directly. Similarly, some women talked about the menopause as if it was something that was happening but they were attempting not to face it. They talked about keeping busy, not thinking about it, and not letting themselves go.

You have to put yourself in order as well because when you go through something like that you become like you are not interested in yourself . . . like you want to let yourself go. You have to occupy your mind. So I think for some women who have nothing to do it must be really terrible for them. They must sit down and think about it and become depressed.

Implicit in several accounts was the idea that if they did stop to find out what 'it' was, there would be negative consequences. Others voiced fears of something vague, difficult, and non-specific happening to them, which was difficult to name or talk about, although concerns about 'letting yourself go', 'becoming depressed', and losing control were indirectly mentioned.

Two women described how by taking HRT they 'wiped out' or 'staved off' the menopause for the time being:

Now it's wiped out, it's a non-event.

Well I feel OK about it, it's what other people desire and need from me that's the difficulty. I've staved off the menopause until my husband catches up with me.

This woman had a young family and a younger husband and felt that going through the menopause did not fit with her current life.

This study illustrates the variation and multidimensional nature of women's accounts of the menopause. Medical language was used

when women initially defined themselves in relation to the menopause, but less so when they spoke about the impact of menopause upon themselves and their lives. In general, the women described the menopause as having little overall impact. They talked of continuation of the self and relief from menstruation. Reproductive decisions, on the whole, were faced earlier in their lives. Women's descriptions of the menopause were complex, varying with material circumstances, for example working environment, hot flushes, past pregnancies, and heavy periods.

As well as dealing with physical changes, women can face an additional task during the menopause—to maintain a positive sense of self amidst menopause and age changes that have unduly negative connotations. Ways of negotiating negative stereotypes of menopause were to see other women as being more prone to problems and by avoiding or staving off the menopause by keeping busy or taking HRT. By 'staving off' the menopause some women may not have the opportunity of finding out whether their experience would in fact conform to their image of it. In this way stereotypes about menopause are easily maintained. In order to demystify the menopause it might be helpful to promote language that is more specific and discriminates between different aspects of the process. For example, the women described hot flushes, menstrual changes, and reproductive changes quite separately. Several women commented that the menopause is still taboo and that few opportunities exist at this stage of life to discuss feelings and experiences in depth. Groups for middle-aged women, which could take place as part of health education strategies, can provide a place for discussion of social and cultural meanings of the menopause and to examine their impact upon one's experience of this stage of life.[23] Such groups might help to develop common understandings, to acknowledge differences between women, and to reinforce challenges to stereotyped images that the middle-aged women in this study voiced in their accounts.

Studies of decision making in relation to hormonal treatments

HRT is being increasingly promoted for the prevention of osteoporosis and cardiovascular disease, as well as for relief of hot flushes and, more recently, for improvements in quality of life. In order to derive long-term health benefits from HRT, at least five years' use is generally recommended.[24] In the medical literature 'compliance' with HRT is regarded as low in terms of both uptake and adherence rates, particularly in the UK, where approximately 15% of 45–55-year-old women currently use HRT. Reasons for low uptake include not wanting to take medication, having menstrual periods, and fears of risks and side-effects. It has been assumed that with

appropriate information and reassurance uptake and adherence would increase.[25] However, an educational model that neglects health beliefs is likely to be overly simplistic. In general, women are more likely than doctors to see the menopause as a normal developmental phase of life, whereas doctors are more likely to see it as a disease-like process.[26] One study of women's attitudes found that promotion of HRT was considered of low priority compared with other health concerns.[27] In a qualitative British study of decision making about HRT, women tended to prefer not to take medication for what they regarded as a 'natural process' unless they had current symptoms, such as hot flushes, and thus appeared, in general, to be using different criteria from health professionals when making decisions about HRT use.[28] This may partly explain why some women report dissatisfaction with medical consultations about the menopause and HRT.[29] The women in the study were also influenced by their doctors' views about HRT. Given that doctors have been found to be uncertain about the balance of costs and benefits of HRT in the long term,[30] and that gynaecologists and general practitioners show little agreement on the prescription of HRT,[31] the information women receive is likely to be variable.

In a detailed study of women's intentions to take HRT, Quine and Rubin[32] found that intention to use HRT was most strongly predicted by having positive beliefs about the benefits of HRT, by the beliefs of significant others (partner, friends, doctor), and by beliefs that they had the resources to negotiate taking HRT with their doctors and that few impediments to taking it exist.

This research points to a need for balanced information and the opportunity to discuss the relative costs and benefits and possible health risks, as well as the woman's values and preferences. In addition, health professionals need to be aware of their own beliefs and values and their possible impact upon the way that information is provided. Decision making about HRT is a complex process that involves estimating future possible health risks and the likely benefits of medical or other interventions. In a recent study we examined women's perceptions of the likelihood that they might develop health problems such as osteoporosis, cardiovascular disease, and breast cancer in the future. They were asked to repeat the estimation imagining that they had taken HRT for 5 years. Overall, women's estimation concurred with population risk statistics, but women were conservative about the perceived preventative effects of HRT, believing it to prevent osteoporosis, but not cardiovascular disease.[33]

Research is also being developed to evaluate ways to empower women for informed decision making during consultations, for example using leaflets, interviews, and videos, in order to overcome barriers such as lack of information, the stigma of the menopause, and differing agendas, gender differences, and power relationships between women and health professionals.[34,35]

Psychological interventions

Psychological interventions include provision of health education and treatments for vasomotor symptoms and for psychological problems reported during the menopause.

In a prospective study the effects of providing 45-year-old women with two health education workshops were examined; these included discussion and provision of balanced information in relation to expectations of menopause, self-help, and medical treatments, and advice about stress reduction and increasing health-related behaviours.[23] Following the intervention, and at 18 months and 5 years later, the intervention group had significantly greater knowledge of the menopause and treatment than a control group who did not receive the intervention.[36] They also had fewer negative beliefs about the menopause at follow-up. Although there were no significant changes in health-related behaviours, there was a strong trend for the health education group to increase levels of exercise.

Despite the prevalence of vasomotor symptoms, it is only recently that psychological treatment studies have been carried out. There are considerable cultural differences in hot flush reporting, but even within Western cultures the experience of hot flushes has proven highly variable when site, frequency, duration, and intensity have been studied. A range of emotional reactions have been reported including embarrassment, panic, feelings of suffocation, and precipitants have been identified such as hot drinks, alcohol, external heat, and stressful situations, but many flushing episodes are described as spontaneous.[37,38] Gannon *et al*[39] monitored 10 women and found a positive correlation between hot flushes and stress (daily hassles) for half the sample.

Approximately 10–15% of women with hot flushes describe them as problematic, largely because of physical discomfort, disruption of sleep, and social embarrassment.[40] Hot flushes and night sweats are the main reason given for seeking medical help during the menopause. The frequency of hot flushes appears to be difficult to predict and was not associated with sociodemographic variables in a recent study. However, women who viewed their flushes as problematic tended to report higher levels of anxiety and depressed mood and lower self-esteem.[40] Hormone replacement therapy is an effective and commonly recommended treatment for hot flushes. However, in view of the possible relationship between hot flush reporting and stress, psychological interventions have been developed that include behavioural treatments,[41] particularly deep breathing and relaxation.[42] In a recent study a cognitive-behavioural intervention, including relaxation, was found to be as effective as HRT in reducing hot flush frequency.[43] This treatment involved four out-patient sessions with a clinical psychologist, during which time vasomotor symptoms were monitored, exacerbators and precipitating factors identified, and stress management was taught. Women discussed ways of dealing with hot flushes using cognitive behavioural approaches and also attempted to reduce stress in their lives. Those receiving the psychological treatment also reported lowered anxiety ratings after treatment. Further research is needed to examine the potent factors within these treatments.

Psychological therapies, such as cognitive behaviour therapy (CBT), are also likely to be helpful for women who attend clinics with emotional problems. CBT has been shown to be effective in the treatment of depression and anxiety for people seeking help from general practitioners or psychiatric services. Few studies have focused specifically on the psychological treatment of women seeking help from menopause clinics. In a pilot study, we compared a problem-solving group treatment (based on cognitive-behavioural principles) with a waiting list control condition for middle-aged women in general practice and found significant reductions in depression and anxiety following treatment compared with the control group.[44] Individual[45] or group therapy[44] might provide a useful forum to help women to clarify the causes of distress in their lives and seek appropriate solutions. Further research is needed to examine the needs and most effective treatment of women attending menopause clinics who experience both emotional and physical problems.

Conclusions

The investigation of psychological aspects of the menopause has broadened in focus during the past century, from a pathological view of menopause as a prime cause of distress and depression, to a consideration of the psychological aspects of a range of variables, such as perceptions of menopause, help-seeking behaviour and treatment decision-making. With methodological improvements in epidemiological studies, evidence for a less negative view of the menopause transition has accumulated. Nevertheless, some women who seek help are depressed, and careful consideration is needed to offer a choice of treatments that address psychosocial as well as health needs.

The application of psychological theoretical models can facilitate understanding of women's help-seeking behaviour in relation to HRT and other treatments, and the development of psychological treatments can help women to deal with vasomotor symptoms, as well as anxiety and depression during this life stage.

References

1. Deutsch H. *The Psychology of Women*, vol 2. New York: Grune & Stratton, 1945.

2. Krafft-Ebing R von. Uber Imesin in Klimakterium. *Psychiatry* 1877; **34**: 407.

3. Showalter E. *The Female Malady*. London: Virago, 1987.

4. Nicol-Smith L. Causality, menopause and depression: a critical review of the literature. *BMJ* 1996; **313**: 1229–1232.

5. Matthews KA, Wing RR, Kuller LH. Influences of natural menopause on psychological characteristics and symptoms of middle-aged healthy women. *J Consult & Clinical Psychol* 1990; **58**: 345–363.

6. Kaufert PA, Gilbert P, Tate R. The Manitoba Project; a re-examination of the relationship between menopause and depression. *Maturitas* 1992; **14**(2): 143–156.

7. McKinlay SM, Brambilla DJ, Posner J. The normal menopause transition. *Maturitas* 1992; **14**(2): 103–116.

8. Dennerstein L. In pursuit of happiness: well-being during the menopausal transition. In: Berg G, Hammer M, eds. *The Modern Management of the Menopause: A Perspective for the 21st Century*. London: Parthenon, 1993.

9. Utian W. Current status of menopause and postmenopausal estrogen therapy. *Obstet Gynecol Surv* 1997; **32**: 193.

10. Porter M, Penney GC, Russell D *et al.* A population based survey of women's experience of the menopause. *Br J Obstet Gynaecol* 1996; **103**: 1025–1028.

11. Hunter MS. The S.E. England longitudinal study of the climacteric and postmenopause. *Maturitas* 1992; **14**(2): 117–126.

12. Bebbington P. The origins of sex differences in depressive disorder: bridging the gap. *Int Rev Psychiatr* 1996; **8**: 295–332.

13. Hunter MS, O'Dea I, Anjos S. Life satisfaction, health concerns and health related quality of life in mid-aged men and women. *Climacteric* 1990; **2**: 131–140.

14. Flint M. The menopause: reward or punishment. *Psychosomatics* 1975; **16**: 161–163.

15. Greene JG. Constructing a standard climacteric scale. *Maturitas* 1998; **29**: 25–31.

16. Hunter MS. The Women's Health Questionnaire: a measure of mid-aged women's emotional and physical health. *Psychol Health* 1990; **7**: 45–54.

17. Alder E. The Blatt–Kupperman menopausal index: a critique. *Maturitas* 1998; **29**: 19–24.

18. Ballinger S. Psychosocial stress and symptoms of menopause: a comparative study of menopause clinic patients and non-patients. *Maturitas* 1985; **7**: 315–327.

19. Hay A, Bancroft J, Johnstone E. Affective symptoms in women attending a menopause clinic. *Br J Psychiatr* 1994; **164**: 513–516.

20. Hunter MS, Marsh MS, Whitehead I. Psychological factors influence help-seeking from menopause clinics. *J Psychosom Obstet Gynaecol* (in press)

21. Hunter MS, O'Dea I. Menopause: bodily changes and multiple meanings. In: Ussher JM, ed. *Body Talk: The Material and Discursive Regulation of Sexuality, Madness and Reproduction.* London: Routledge, 1997, 199–222.

22. Potter J, Wetherell M. *Discourse and Social Psychology: Beyond Attitudes and Beliefs.* London: Sage, 1987.

23. Liao KLM, Hunter MS. Preparation for the menopause: prospective evaluation of a health education intervention for mid-aged women. *Maturitas* 1998; **29**: 215–224.

24. Coope J. *Hormone Replacement Therapy.* London: RCGP, 1989.

25. Sinclair HK, Bond CM, Taylor RJ. Hormone replacement therapy: a study of women's knowledge and attitudes. *Br J Gen Pract* 1993; **43**: 365–370.

26. Leiblum SR, Swartzman LS. Women's attitudes about the menopause: an update. *Maturitas* 1986; **81**: 47–56.

27. Griffiths F. Women's health concerns. Is the promotion of hormone replacement therapy for prevention important for women? *Family Pract* 1995; **12**: 54–59.

28. Hunter MS, O'Dea I, Britten N. Decision making and hormone replacement therapy: a qualitative study. *Soc Sci Med* 1997; **45**: 1541–1548.

29. Hibbard JH, Sampson SE. Enhancing women's partnership with health providers in hormone replacement therapy decision making: research and practice directions. *J Women Ageing* 1993; **5**: 17–29.

30. Wilkes HC, Meade TW. Hormone replacement therapy in general practice: a survey of doctors in the MRC's general practice research framework. *BMJ* 1991; **302**: 1317–1320.

31. Norman SG, Studd JW. A survey of views on hormone replacement therapy. *Br J Obstet Gynaecol* 1994; **101**: 879–887.

32. Quine L, Rubin R. Attitude, subjective norm,

and perceived behavioural control as predictors of women's intentions to take hormone replacement therapy. *Br J Health Psychol* 1997; **2**: 199–216.

33. Hunter MS, O'Dea I. Perception of future health risks in mid-aged women and men: estimates with and without hypothetical behavioural changes and hormone replacement therapy. *Maturitas* 1999; **33**: 37–43.

34. Hampson SE, Hibbard JH. Cross-talk about the menopause: enhancing interactions about menopause and hormone replacement therapy. *Patient Educ Counsell* 1996; **27**: 177–184.

35. Rothert M, Padonu G, Holmes-Rovner M *et al*. Menopausal women as decision makers in health care. *Exp Gerontol* 1994; **29**: 463–468.

36. Hunter MS, O'Dea I. An evaluation of a health education intervention for mid-aged women in primary care: five year follow-up of effects upon knowledge, impact of menopause and health. *Patient Educ Counsell* 1999; **38**: 249–255.

37. Voda AM. Climacteric hot flush. *Maturitas* 1981; **3**: 73–90.

38. Kronenberg F. Hot flushes: epidemiology and physiology. *Ann NY Acad Sci* 1990; **592**: 52–86.

39. Gannon L, Hansel S, Goodwin J. Correlates of menopausal hot flushes. *J Behav Med* 1987; **10**: 277–285.

40. Hunter MS, Liao KLM. A psychological analysis of menopausal hot flushes. *Br J Clin Psychol* 1995; **34**: 589–599.

41. Stevenson DW, Delprato DJ. Multiple component self control programme for menopausal hot flashes. *J Behav Ther Exp Psychiatry* 1983; **14**: 137–140.

42. Freedman RR, Woodward S. Behavioural treatment of menopausal hot flushes: evaluation by ambulatory monitoring. *Am J Obstet Gynecol* 1992; **167**: 436–439.

43. Hunter MS, Liao KLM. Evaluation of a four-session cognitive-behavioural intervention for menopausal hot flushes. *Br J Health Psychol* 1996; **1**: 113–125.

44. Hunter MS, Liao KLM. Problem-solving groups for midaged women in general practice: a pilot study. *J Infant Reprod Psychol* 1995; **13**: 147–151.

45. Greene JG, Hart DM. The evaluation of a psychological treatment programme for menopausal women. *Maturitas* 1987; **9**: 1, 41–48.

Oestrogen and the bladder

Andrew Hextall, Linda Cardozo

3

Introduction

Evidence from both animal and human studies suggests that oestrogen has an important effect on the female lower urinary tract throughout adult life. Sex steroid receptors have been identified throughout the brain, in the pontine micturition centre, and in the bladder, urethra, and pelvic floor. It is therefore not surprising that fluctuations in the circulating level of oestrogen and progesterone are thought to be responsible for changes in the prevalence of urinary symptoms and the results of urodynamic investigation which occur during the menstrual cycle and in pregnancy. In addition, epidemiological studies have implicated the menopause and subsequent oestrogen deficiency in the aetiology of a number of urogenital complaints, including incontinence, urgency, and recurrent urinary tract infection. Oestrogens have been used widely to treat urinary symptoms in postmenopausal women, but there are relatively few randomized studies, which makes it difficult to draw accurate conclusions about the true efficacy of such treatment. The aim of this chapter is to discuss the role of oestrogen in the pathogenesis and treatment of lower urinary tract disorders.

Action of oestrogen on the female lower urinary tract

For a woman to remain continent urethral pressure must exceed the intravesical pressure at all times except during micturition.[1] This effect is achieved by the complex interaction of neuromuscular factors and the connective tissue supports of the bladder and urethra.

Control of micturition

Sex steroids appear to influence the central neuronal control of micturition and the continence mechanism. Oestrogen receptors are found throughout the brain cortex, limbic system, hippocampus, and cerebellum.[2,3] Recent animal studies have also shown that androgen receptors are present in the pontine micturition centre[4] and in the preoptic area of the hypothalamus, an area of the forebrain which may play an important role in the initiation of micturition. However, the exact type and distribution of sex steroid receptors in the human micturition pathways and their importance in the control of continence are at present unknown.

Bladder

Oestrogen receptors are not found in the transitional epithelium of the bladder apart from in areas of the trigone which have undergone squamous metaplasia.[5] However,

oestrogen has a direct (non-genomic) effect on detrusor function through modifications in muscarinic receptors[6,7] and inhibition of movement of extracellular calcium ions into muscle cells.[8] Animal studies have shown that oophorectomy alters the pressure flow characteristics of micturition in the female rat.[9] This effect may be only partly reversed by oestrogen supplementation and is possibly age dependent. It is at present unknown whether similar effects occur in humans. Oestradiol reduces the amplitude and frequency of spontaneous rhythmic contractions, which have been associated with detrusor instability,[10] and in vivo oestrogen pretreatment reduces the contractile response of isolated rat detrusor muscle.[11] The sensory threshold of the human bladder may also be raised by oestrogen supplementation.[12]

Urethra

Oestrogen receptors are consistently expressed in the squamous epithelium of the proximal and distal urethra, vagina, and pubococcygeous muscle of the pelvic floor.[5,13–15] A number of authors have shown that oestrogen increases urethral closure pressure and improves pressure transmission to the proximal urethra, effects that probably occur by a combination of different mechanisms.[16–19] In response to oestrogen there is an increase in cell cycle activity and an improved 'maturation index' of the urethral epithelium,[20–22] with similar changes also occurring in the vagina of postmenopausal women.[23,24] Alterations in urinary cytology during the menstrual cycle are comparable to those seen in vaginal cytology,[25] changes that can also be identified in the urinary sediment following treatment with oestrogens.[26]

The vasodilatory effects of oestrogens which occur in the systemic and cerebral circulations also take place in the female urethra.[27–29] Versi and Cardozo[30] have shown that vascular pulsations seen on urethral pressure profilometry (UPP), secondary to blood flow in the urethral submucosa and urethral sphincter, increase in size in response to oestrogen. Attempts have been made to quantify changes in urethral blood flow in response to oestrogen therapy using Doppler ultrasound.[31] Unfortunately, difficulties in imaging the same vessel repeatedly and natural variation in blood flow through pelvic vessels limit the reproducibility of the technique.

Connective tissue metabolism and production of collagen are stimulated by oestrogens, thus reversing the reduction in total vaginal and periurethral collagen which is associated with genuine stress incontinence and genitourinary prolapse.[32–34] Recent evidence suggests that these conditions are both associated with a systemic change in collagenase activity.[35] However, it is unclear whether prophylactic treatment with hormone replacement is sufficient to prevent their development, particularly in view of the fact that both have multifactorial aetiology.

Oestrogen and urinary symptoms

Cyclical variations in the level of sex steroids during the menstrual cycle may lead to both symptomatic and urodynamic changes. Approximately 40% of premenopausal women with regular periods complain that their urinary symptoms change with the menstrual cycle, with the time just before a period identified as the most bothersome (*Fig. 3.1*).[36] The prevalence of detrusor instability on cystometry also increases significantly with time from the last menstrual period and may reflect increases in the circulating level of progesterone following ovulation. There also appears to be a relationship between changes in serum oestradiol and alterations in the functional urethral length measured with urethral pressure profilometry.[37] Many women complain of urinary symptoms during pregnancy which are only in part due to an increase in urine output and pressure effects from the gravid uterus.[38–40] The prevalence of detrusor instability antenatally is significantly greater than that found postpartum,[41] suggesting a possible hormonal effect also thought to be mediated through progesterone.

Progesterone receptors are expressed inconsistently in the lower urinary tract and

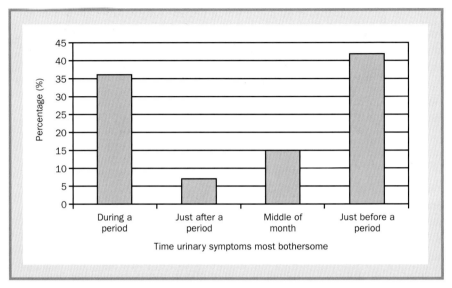

Figure 3.1
Time urinary symptoms are most bothersome in relation to the menstrual cycle.[36] Percentage of positive responses of 55/133 women with a regular cycle (not on the combined contraceptive pill or other hormonal therapy) who indicated that their urinary symptoms changed during the menstrual cycle.

may be dependent on the oestrogen status of the woman.[5,42] Unfortunately, there are very little data on the physiological effects of progesterone outside pregnancy,[43] but in general progestogens have an adverse effect on the bladder and urethra. Elliot and Castleden[44] have shown that progesterone antagonizes the inhibitory effect of oestradiol on rat detrusor muscle contractions. Clinically, progestogens are associated with an increase in irritative bladder symptoms[45,46] and urinary leakage in those women with incontinence taking hormone replacement therapy.[47] However, progestogens do not appear to alter significantly the urethral pressure profile of continent women.[48] Androgen receptors are found in both the female bladder and urethra, but their role is at present unclear.[49]

Several epidemiological reports have implicated oestrogen deficiency in the aetiology of a number of different urinary complaints. Iosif and Bekassy[50] studied 2200 women aged 61 years and found that 70% of women with incontinence related the onset of their urinary leakage to the time of their final menstrual period. In a survey of 2045 British women aged between 55 and 85 years, Barlow and colleagues[51] showed that urogenital symptoms had affected 48.5% of postmenopausal women at some time and that 11% were currently troubled by individual complaints. Urinary tract symptoms are certainly common following the menopause, with one in five women attending a menopause clinic complaining of severe urgency, and nearly 50% complaining of stress incontinence.[52]

The prevalence of postmenopausal incontinence in the community is thought to be between 16% and 29%.[53–55] Although there are clearly a number of important factors in the pathogenesis of urinary incontinence, there is conflicting evidence regarding the role of the menopause. Thomas and colleagues[56] and Jolleys[53] found the peak prevalence of urinary incontinence in community-dwelling women to occur in the perimenopausal age group. Hilton[57] found a similar pattern of prevalence in hospital practice, with 40% of women referred to a urogynaecology unit aged between 40 and 60 years, with a mean comparable to that of the menopause. Urge incontinence in particular is found more commonly following the menopause[58] with the prevalence appearing to rise in line with increasing years of oestrogen

deficiency (*Fig. 3.2*). However, most studies show that many women develop incontinence at least 10 years before their last period, with Jolleys[53] and Burgio and colleagues[59] finding that significantly more premenopausal women than postmenopausal women were affected. The prevalence of stress incontinence in the community also starts to fall following the menopause, and the increase in urge incontinence and detrusor instability in elderly women may simply be an effect of the ageing process.

There are a number of reasons why oestrogens may be useful for the treatment of lower urinary tract symptoms (*Table 3.1*).

Table 3.1
Mechanisms by which oestrogen may be useful for the treatment of urinary incontinence.

Increased urethral closure pressure

- *Increased urethral cell maturation*
- *Increased urethral blood flow*
- *Increased alpha-adrenergic receptor sensitivity in urethral smooth muscle*

Improved abdominal pressure transmission to proximal urethra
Stimulation of periurethral collagen production
Improved neuronal control of micturition
Increased sensory threshold of the bladder
Improved mood and quality of life
Reduced incidence of urinary tract infection

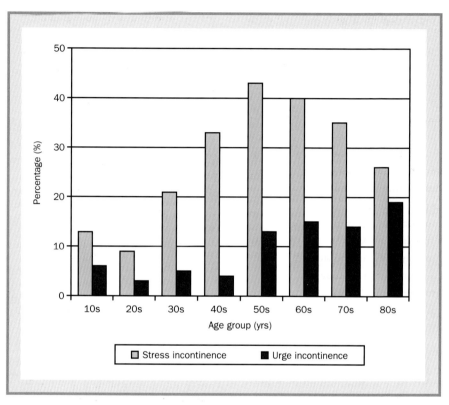

Figure 3.2
Prevalence of the symptoms of stress incontinence and urge incontinence among 1100 Japanese women.[58]

Salmon and colleagues[60] were the first to report the successful use of oestrogens to treat urinary incontinence over 50 years ago. However, it is now well recognized that there is a poor correlation between a woman's symptoms and the subsequent diagnosis following appropriate investigation.[61] Unfortunately, initial trials took place before the widespread introduction of urodynamic studies and therefore almost certainly included women with a number of different pathologies.

Oestrogen for stress incontinence

There are a large number of published studies of oestrogen for the treatment of urinary stress incontinence but most have to be interpreted with caution because they are observational and not randomized, blinded, or controlled. Comparison of the different reports is also difficult because a number of different types of oestrogen have been used with varying doses, routes of administration, and durations of treatment. The concurrent use of progestogens, to prevent endometrial hyperplasia in those women with a uterus, probably also influences success rates.

In an attempt to clarify the situation the Hormones and Urogenital Therapy (HUT) committee has performed a meta-analysis of oestrogens for incontinence.[62] Of 166 articles identified which were published in English between 1969 and 1992, only six were controlled trials and 17 were uncontrolled series. Subjectively, oestrogen was found to produce a significant improvement for all patients and those with genuine stress incontinence, but this may have been because oestrogens improve feelings of well-being and quality of life. Analysis of objective parameters failed to show any reduction in the volume of urine lost compared with pretreatment levels.

Two further studies using oral oestrogen, which were not included in the HUT meta-analysis, have recently been reported. Fantl *et al*[63] performed a randomized trial of 83 hypo-oestrogenic patients with urodynamically proven genuine stress incontinence and/or detrusor instability. Women were treated for 3 months with cyclical conjugated equine oestrogens 0.625 mg and medroxyprogesterone 10 mg or a placebo. At the end of the study period the clinical and quality of life variables had not changed significantly in either group. Although this may have been due to the lack of efficacy of the oestrogen prescribed, the mixed pathology of some of the women and the concurrent use of progestogens make it difficult to draw any firm conclusions. Jackson and co-workers[64] treated 67 postmenopausal women with genuine stress incontinence or mixed incontinence with oestradiol valerate 2 mg or placebo daily for 6 months in a double-blind, placebo-controlled study. Six of the 33 women randomized to receive oestradiol experienced breakthrough bleeding during the trial and were subsequently treated with an additional monthly progestogen. Although this is one of the largest studies yet reported, with the longest duration of treatment, there were again no significant changes in the subjective or objective outcome measures. It should be noted that, similar to other reports, the mean age of the women treated was 63 years. It is possible that irreversible changes in the lower urinary tract may already have taken place in this age group, with only those women in the perimenopausal years likely to benefit from this form of treatment.

Alpha-adrenergic receptors in the urethral sphincter are sensitized by oestrogens, which helps to maintain muscular tone.[65] Several studies have utilized this effect and shown that oestrogen may be a useful treatment for stress incontinence if given with alpha-adrenergic agents. Beisland and colleagues[66] and Hilton and colleagues[67] used oestrogen in combination with phenylpropanolamine (50 mg twice daily) and found both subjective and objective benefits which were greater than for either treatment given alone. This type of therapy may be particularly useful for women with mild stress incontinence or for cases not suitable for surgery.

Oestrogens for the 'urge syndrome'

There are a number of causes of urinary frequency and urgency in postmenopausal women (*Table 3.2*) and investigation is often required to make an accurate diagnosis. In several studies oestrogen has been used to treat urgency and urge incontinence regardless of the underlying pathology and in others even women who initially developed their symptoms many years before the menopause have been included in the assessment. Perhaps for these reasons very few trials have shown oestrogen to be of benefit for this condition, although again there is a lack of large, randomized, controlled studies with a long duration of treatment from which to make conclusions. In addition, a large placebo effect occurs in the treatment of this

condition and therefore trials involving small numbers of patients need to be interpreted with caution.[68,69]

In a recent double-blind multicentre study 64 postmenopausal women with the 'urge syndrome' were randomized to treatment with oral oestriol 3 mg daily or placebo for 3 months.[70] Urodynamic studies were performed at baseline and compliance was confirmed by a significant improvement in the maturation index of vaginal epithelial cells in the active but not the placebo group. Oestriol

Table 3.2
Common causes of urinary frequency and urgency in postmenopausal women.

Systemic
• Diabetes mellitus
• Diuretic therapy
Psychosocial
• Excessive fluid intake
• Habit/anxiety
Urogynaecological
• Detrusor instability
• Sensory urgency
• Low bladder compliance
• Voiding difficulty
• Bladder mucosal abnormality, e.g. cystitis, papilloma, carcinoma
• Urethral lesion, e.g. urethritis, diverticulum, caruncle
• Urogenital prolapse
• Sexual intercourse
• Urinary tract infection
• Postmenopausal urogenital atrophy

produced subjective and objective improvements in urinary symptoms, but it was not significantly better than placebo. Sustained-release 25 mg 17β-oestradiol vaginal tablets (Vagifem®, Novo Nordisk, Crawley (West Sussex), UK) or placebo were used by Benness and colleagues to treat 110 postmenopausal women.[71] At the end of the 6 month treatment period the only significant difference between the active and placebo groups was an improvement in the symptom of urgency in the women who had a urodynamic diagnosis of sensory urgency. In these women it was possible that the oestrogen was reversing atrophic changes in the lower urogenital tract rather than treating any underlying bladder pathology.

Oestrogen and urinary tract infection

Urinary tract infections (UTI) occur commonly in women of all ages. This is a particular problem in the elderly, with a reported incidence of 20% in community-dwelling women and sometimes over 50% in institutionalized patients.[72,73] Pathophysiological changes that may account for this increase include impairment of bladder emptying, poor perineal hygiene, and both faecal and urinary incontinence. Alterations in the vaginal flora associated with oestrogen deficiency are also thought to place women at risk of UTI, particularly if they are sexually

active. There is a rise in vaginal pH and fall in the number of lactobacilli, allowing colonization with Gram-negative bacteria that act as uropathogens. However, the exact role of the menopause as an aetiological factor in the development of UTI may have been overstated. Analysis of mid-stream urine specimens (MSU) sent to our hospital from the community indicate that the proportion of positive results increases with age in both men and women, with no specific changes in the rate of infection occurring at or following the menopause.[74]

Oestrogen reverses the microbiological changes in the vaginal flora which occur as a result of the menopause, an effect that enables oestrogen to be used for treatment or prophylaxis. Initial small uncontrolled studies[75–77] using oral or vaginal therapy produced encouraging results. Five randomized studies of oestrogen for this condition have now also been reported (*Table 3.3*).[78–82] In the largest trial to date, Eriksen[82] conducted a multicentre, randomized, open, parallel-group study of 108 postmenopausal women with recurrent, symptomatic, bacteriologically confirmed urinary tract infections. The women were randomly assigned to receive either Estring (2 mg oestradiol; Pharmacia & Upjohn, Uppsala, Sweden) or no oestrogen treatment. After 36 weeks of study the cumulative likelihood of remaining free of infection was 45% in the women with the vaginal ring compared with approximately 20% in the control group. A

Table 3.3
Randomized studies of oestrogen for recurrent urinary tract infections.

Study	Study group	Type of oestrogen	Route of delivery	Duration of therapy	Results
Kjaergaard et al 1990[78]	21 postmenopausal women with recurrent cystitis 10 active group 11 placebo	Oestradiol	Vaginal tablets	5 months	Number of positive cultures not statistically different between the two groups.
Kirkengen et al 1992[79]	40 postmenopausal women with recurrent UTIs 20 active group 20 placebo	Oestriol	Oral	12 weeks	Both oestriol and placebo significantly reduced the incidence of UTIs ($p < 0.05$). After 12 weeks oestriol was significantly more effective than placebo ($p < 0.05$).
Raz and Stamm 1993[80]	93 postmenopausal women with recurrent UTIs 50 active group 43 placebo	Oestriol	Vaginal cream	8 months	Significant reduction in the incidence of UTIs in the group given oestriol compared with placebo ($p < 0.001$).
Cardozo et al 1998[81]	72 postmenopausal women with recurrent UTIs 36 active group 36 placebo	Oestriol	Oral	6 months treatment period with a further 6 months follow-up	Reduction in urinary symptoms and incidence of UTIs in both groups. Oestriol no better than placebo.
Eriksen 1999[82]	108 women with recurrent UTIs 53 active group 55 no treatment	Oestradiol	Estring	36 weeks for the active group; 36 weeks or until first recurrence for the controls	Cumulative likelihood of remaining free of infection was 45% in active group and 20% in control group ($p = 0.008$).

randomized, double-blind, placebo-controlled study of 93 postmenopausal women has also shown that intravaginal oestriol cream reduces the risk of recurrence of urinary tract infection.[80] The incidence of urinary tract infection in the group given oestriol was significantly lower than in women given placebo (0.5 versus 5.9 episodes per patient per year). Changes in the vaginal pH and colonization with lactobacilli were present in the oestriol group only within 1 month of the start of treatment.

The HUT committee has recently reported a systematic review of oestrogen for recurrent UTIs and concluded that vaginal oestrogen administration seems to be effective for this condition.[83] However, it is important to note that although UTI is one of the most common reasons why a woman may present to her doctor, fewer than 400 women have taken part in randomized studies of oestrogen for this condition, and two of the five reported randomized trials[78,81] have failed to demonstrate any advantage of oestrogen over placebo.

Conclusions

Sex steroids have an important physiological effect on the female lower urinary tract, and oestrogen deficiency is associated with a number of urogenital complaints. The use of hormone replacement therapy to treat urinary symptoms has given conflicting and largely disappointing results. When oestrogens are used alone to treat stress incontinence there is no objective improvement in urinary leakage, but they may be useful when given in combination with alpha-adrenergic agonists. Oestrogen supplementation given locally or orally may improve the irritative symptoms of urinary frequency and urgency, possibly by reversing urogenital atrophy, but most studies have failed to show an effect greater than that of placebo. Treatment may need to be given for several weeks or even months for maximum efficacy but the optimal route of delivery and duration of therapy remain to be determined. Oestrogen appears to be of benefit for prophylaxis against recurrent urinary tract infection, particularly if it is administered vaginally.

References

1. Abrams P, Blaivas JG, Stanton SL *et al.* The standardisation of terminology of lower urinary tract dysfunction. *Br J Obstet Gynaecol* 1990; 97: 1–16.

2. Maggi A, Perez J. Role of female gonadal hormones in the CNS. *Life Sci* 1985; 37: 893–906.

3. Smith SS. Hormones, mood and neurobiology—a summary. In: Berg G, Hammar M, eds. *The Modern Management of the Menopause.* Carnforth, UK: Parthenon, 1993, 204.

4. Blok BFM, Holstege G. Androgen receptor immunoreactive neurons in the hypothalamic preoptic area project to the pontine

micturition centre in the male cat. *Neurourol Urodyn* 1998; **17**: 404–405.

5.   Blakeman PJ, Hilton P, Bulmer JN. Mapping oestrogen and progesterone receptors throughout the female lower urinary tract. *Neurourol Urodyn* 1996; **15**: 324–325.

6.   Shapiro E. Effect of oestrogens on the weight and muscarinic receptor density of the rabbit bladder and urethra. *J Urol* 1986; **135**: 1084–1087.

7.   Batra S, Anderson KE. Oestrogen-induced changes in muscarinic receptor density and contractile responses in the female rat urinary bladder. *Acta Physiol Scand* 1989; **137**: 135–141.

8.   Elliott RA, Castleden CM, Miodrag A *et al.* The direct effects of diethylstilboestrol and nifedipine on the contractile responses of isolated human and rat detrusor muscles. *Eur J Clin Pharmacol* 1992; **43**: 149–155.

9.   Diep N, Yokota T, Soo Choo M *et al.* Effect of estrogen supplementation of ovariectomized rats on micturition. *Neurourol Urodyn* 1998; **17**: 405–406.

10. Shenfield OZ, Blackmore PF, Morgan CW *et al.* Rapid effects of estradiol and progesterone on tone and spontaneous rhythmic contractions of the rabbit bladder. *Neurourol Urodyn* 1998; **17**: 408–409.

11. Elliott RA, Castleden CM, Miodrag A. The effect of *in vivo* oestrogen pretreatment on the contractile response of rat isolated detrusor muscle. *Br J Pharmacol* 1992; **107**: 766–770.

12. Fantl JA, Wyman JF, Anderson RL *et al.* Postmenopausal urinary incontinence: comparison between non-estrogen and estrogen supplemented women. *Obstet Gynecol* 1988; **71**: 823–828.

13. Iosif CS, Batra S, Ek A. Estrogen receptors in the human female lower urinary tract. *Am J Obstet Gynecol* 1981; **141**: 817–820.

14. Ingelman-Sundberg A, Rosen J, Gustafsson SA. Cytosol oestrogen receptors in urogenital tissues in stress incontinent women. *Acta Obstet Gynecol Scand* 1981; **60**: 585–586.

15. Smith P. Estrogens and the urogential tract. *Acta Obstet Gynecol Scand* 1993; **72** (suppl): 1–26.

16. Rud T. The effects of estrogens and gestogens on the urethral pressure profile in urinary continent and stress incontinent women. *Acta Obstet Gynecol Scand* 1980; **59**: 265–270.

17. Hilton P, Stanton SL. The use of intravaginal oestrogen cream in genuine stress incontinence. *Br J Obstet Gynaecol* 1983; **90**: 940–944.

18. Bhatia NN, Bergman A, Karram MM *et al.* Effects of oestrogen on urethral function in women with urinary incontinence. *Am J Obstet Gynecol* 1989; **160**: 176–181.

19. Karram MM, Yeko TR, Sauer MV *et al.* Urodynamic changes following hormone replacement therapy in women with premature ovarian failure. *Obstet Gynecol* 1989; **74**: 208–211.

20. Bergman A, Karram MM, Bhatia NN. Changes in urethral cytology following estrogen administration. *Gynecol Obstet Invest* 1990; **29**: 211–213.

21. Blakeman PJ, Hilton P, Bulmer JN. Oestrogen status and cell cycle activity in the female lower urinary tract. *Neurourol Urodyn* 1996; **15**: 325–326.

22. Samsioe G, Jansson I, Meelstrom D *et al.* Occurrence, nature and treatment of urinary incontinence in a 70 year old female population. *Maturitas* 1985; 7: 335–342.

23. Smith PJB. The effect of oestrogens on bladder function. In: Campbell S, ed. *Management of the Menopause and Postmenopausal Years.* Lancaster: MTP Press, 1976, 291–298.

24. Semmens JP, Tsai CC, Semmens EC *et al.* Effects of estrogen therapy on vaginal physiology during the menopause. *Obstet Gynecol* 1985; **66**: 15–18.

25. McCallin PF, Taylor ES, Whitehead RW. A study of the changes in the urinary sediment during the menstrual cycle. *Am J Obstet Gynecol* 1950; **60**: 64–74.

26. Soloman C, Panagotopoulos P, Oppenheim A. The use of urinary sediment as an aid in endocrinological disorders in the female. *Am J Obstet Gynecol* 1958; **76**: 56–60.

27. Ganger KF, Vyas S, Whitehead RW *et al.* Pulsatility index in the internal carotid artery in relation to transdermal oestradiol and time since the menopause. *Lancet* 1991; **338**: 839–842.

28. Jackson S, Vyas S. A double-blind, placebo controlled study of postmenopausal oestrogen replacement therapy and carotid artery pulsatility index. *Br J Obstet Gynaecol* 1998; **105**: 408–412.

29. Penotti M, Farina M, Sironi L *et al.* Long term effects of postmenopausal hormone replacement therapy on pulsatility index of internal carotid and middle cerebral arteries. *Menopause* 1997; **4**: 101–104.

30. Versi E, Cardozo LD. Urethral instability: diagnosis based on variations in the maximum urethral pressure in normal climacteric women. *Neurourol Urodyn* 1986; **5**: 535–541.

31. Jackson S, McDonnell C, James M *et al.* Is postmenopausal urethral blood flow affected by hormone replacement therapy? A placebo controlled pilot study. *Neurourol Urodyn* 1997; **16**: 352–353.

32. Jackson S, Avery N, Shepherd A *et al.* The effect of oestradiol on vaginal collagen in postmenopausal women with stress urinary incontinence. *Neurourol Urodyn* 1996; **15**: 327–328.

33. James M, Avery N, Jackson S *et al.* The pathophysiological changes of vaginal tissue in women with stress urinary incontinence: a controlled trial. *Neurourol Urodyn* 1999; **18**: 283–284.

34. James M, Avery N, Jackson S *et al.* The biochemical profile of vaginal tissue in women with genitourinary prolapse: a controlled trial. *Neurourol Urodyn* 1999; **18**: 284–285.

35. Kushner L, Chen Y, Desautel M *et al.* Collagenase activity is elevated in conditioned media from fibroblasts of women with pelvic floor weakening. *Neurourol Urodyn* 1999; **18**: 282–283.

36. Hextall A, Bidmead J, Cardozo L *et al.* Hormonal influences on the human female lower urinary tract: a prospective evaluation of the effects of the menstrual cycle on symptomatology and the results of urodynamic investigation. *Neurourol Urodyn* 1999; **18**: 363–364.

37. Van Geelen JM, Doesburg WH, Thomas CMG. Urodynamic studies in the normal menstrual cycle: the relationship between hormonal changes during the menstrual cycle and the urethral pressure profile. *Am J Obstet Gynecol* 1981; **141**: 384–392.

38. Stanton SL, Kerr-Wilson R, Harris VG. The incidence of urological symptoms in normal pregnancy. *Br J Obstet Gynaecol* 1980; **87**: 897–900.

39. Cutner A, Carey A, Cardozo LD. Lower urinary tract symptoms in early pregnancy. *J Obstet Gynaecol* 1992; **12**: 75–78.

40. Chaliha C, Kalia V, Stanton SL *et al.* What

does pregnancy and delivery do to bladder function? A urodynamic viewpoint. *Neurourol Urodyn* 1998; **17**: 415–416.

41.   Cutner A. The lower urinary tract in pregnancy. MD thesis, University of London, London, 1993.

42.   Batra SC, Iosif CS. Progesterone receptors in the female lower urinary tract. *J Urol* 1987; **138**: 1301–1304.

43.   Swift SE, Ostergard DR. Effects of progesterone on the urinary tract. *Int Urogynecol J* 1993; **4**: 232–236.

44.   Elliott RA, Castleden CM. Effect of progestogens and oestrogens on the contractile response of rat detrusor muscle to electrical field stimulation. *Clinical Science* 1994; **87**: 342.

45.   Burton G, Cardozo LD, Abdalla H *et al.* The hormonal effects on the lower urinary tract in 282 women with premature ovarian failure. *Neurourol Urodyn* 1992; **10**: 319.

46.   Cutner A, Burton G, Cardozo LD *et al.* Does progesterone cause an irritable bladder? *Int Urogynecol J* 1993; **4**: 261.

47.   Benness C, Gangar K, Cardozo LD *et al.* Do progestogens exacerbate urinary incontinence in women on HRT? *Neurourol Urodyn* 1991; **10**: 316–318.

48.   Raz S, Ziegler M, Laine M. The effect of progesterone on the adrenergic receptors of the urethra. *Br J Urol* 1973; **45**: 131–135.

49.   Blakeman PJ, Hilton P, Bulmer JN. Androgen receptors in the female lower urinary tract. *Int Urogynecol J* 1997; **8**: S54.

50.   Iosif CS, Bekassey Z. Prevalence of genito-urinary symptoms in the late menopause. *Acta Obstet Gynecol Scand* 1984; **63**: 257–260.

51.   Barlow DH, Cardozo LD, Francis RM *et al.*

Urogenital ageing and its effect on sexual health in older British women. *Br J Obstet Gynaecol* 1997; **104**: 87–91.

52.   Cardozo LD, Tapp A, Versi E. The lower urinary tract in peri- and postmenopausal women. In: Samsioe G, Bonne Erickson P, eds. *The Urogenital Oestrogen Deficiency Syndrome.* Bagsverd, Denmark: Novo Industri, 1987, 10–17.

53.   Jolleys JV. Reported prevalence of urinary incontinence in a general practice. *BMJ* 1988; **296**: 1300–1302.

54.   Rekers H, Drogendijk AC, Valkenburg H *et al.* Urinary incontinence in women from 35 to 79 years of age: prevalence and consequences. *Eur J Obstet Gynecol Reprod Biol* 1992; **43**: 229–234.

55.   Vetter NJ, Jones DA, Victor CR. Urinary incontinence in the elderly at home. *Lancet* 1981; **2**: 1275–1277.

56.   Thomas TM, Plymat KR, Blannin J *et al.* Prevalence of urinary incontinence. *BMJ* 1980; **281**: 1243–1245.

57.   Hilton P. Urethral pressure measurement by micro transducer: observations on the methodology, the pathophysiology of stress incontinence and the effects of treatment in the female. MD thesis, University of Newcastle upon Tyne, Newcastle upon Tyne, 1983.

58.   Kondo A, Kato K, Saito M *et al.* Prevalence of hand washing incontinence in females in comparison with stress and urge incontinence. *Neurourol Urodyn* 1990; **9**: 330–331.

59.   Burgio KL, Matthews KA, Engel B. Prevalence, incidence and correlates of urinary incontinence in healthy, middle aged women. *J Urol* 1991; **146**: 1255–1259.

60.   Salmon UL, Walter RI, Gast SH. The use of

estrogen in the treatment of dysuria and incontinence in postmenopausal women. *Am J Obstet Gynecol* 1941; **14**: 23–31.

61. Jarvis GJ, Hall S, Stamp S *et al*. An assessment of urodynamic investigation in incontinent women. *Br J Obstet Gynaecol* 1980; **87**: 184–190.

62. Fantl JA, Cardozo LD, McClish DK *et al*. Estrogen therapy in the management of urinary incontinence in postmenopausal women: a meta-analysis. *Obstet Gynecol* 1994; **83**: 12–18.

63. Fantl JA, Bump RC, Robinson D *et al*. Efficacy of estrogen supplementation in the treatment of urinary incontinence. *Obstet Gynecol* 1996; **88**: 745–749.

64. Jackson S, Shepherd A, Brookes S *et al*. The effect of oestrogen supplementation on post-menopausal urinary stress incontinence: a double-blind, placebo-controlled trial. *Br J Obstet Gynaecol* 1999; **106**: 711–718.

65. Screiter F, Fuchs P, Stockamp K. Estrogenic sensitivity of alpha receptors in the urethral musculature. *Urol Int* 1976; **31**: 13–19.

66. Beisland HO, Fossberg E, Moer A *et al*. Urethral insufficiency in postmenopausal females: treatment with phenylpropanolamine and estriol separately and in combination. *Urol Int* 1984; **39**: 216.

67. Hilton P, Tweddel AL, Mayne C. Oral and intravaginal estrogens alone and in combination with alpha adrenergic stimulation in genuine stress incontinence. *Int Urogynecol J* 1990; **12**: 80–86.

68. Walter S, Wolf H, Barlebo H *et al*. Urinary incontinence in postmenopausal women treated with oestrogen. *Urol Int* 1978; **33**: 143.

69. Samsioe G, Jansson I, Mellstrom D *et al*. Urinary incontinence in 75-year-old women. Effects of estriol. *Acta Obstet Gynecol Scand* 1985; suppl 93: 57.

70. Cardozo LD, Rekers H, Tapp A *et al*. Oestriol in the treatment of postmenopausal urgency: a multicentre study. *Maturitas* 1993; **18**: 47–53.

71. Benness C, Wise BG, Cutner A *et al*. Does low dose vaginal estradiol improve frequency and urgency in postmenopausal women? *Int Urogynecol J* 1992; **3**: 281.

72. Sandford JP. Urinary tract symptoms and infection. *Ann Rev Med* 1975; **26**: 485–498.

73. Boscia JA, Kaye D. Asymptomatic bacteria in the elderly. *Infect Dis Clin North Am* 1987; **1**: 893–903.

74. Hextall A, Hooper R, Cardozo LD *et al*. Urogenital ageing and the risk of urinary tract infection. 23rd Annual Meeting, International Urogynaecology Association, Buenos Aires, Argentina, 1998.

75. Parsons CL, Schmidt JD. Control of recurrent lower urinary tract infections in postmenopausal women. *J Urol* 1982; **128**: 1224–1226.

76. Brandberg A, Mellstrom D, Samsioe G. Low dose oral oestriol treatment in elderly women with urogenital infections. *Acta Obstet Gynecol Scand* 1987; **140**: 33–38.

77. Privette M, Cade R, Peterson J *et al*. Prevention of recurrent urinary tract infections in postmenopausal women. *Nephron* 1988; **50**: 24–27.

78. Kjaergaard B, Walter S, Knudsen A *et al*. Treatment with low dose vaginal estradiol in postmenopausal women. A double blind controlled trial. *Ugeskr Laeger* 1990; **152**: 658–659.

79. Kirkengen AL, Anderson P, Gjersoe E *et al.* Oestriol in the prophylactic treatment of recurrent urinary tract infections in postmenopausal women. *Scan J Prim Health Care* 1992; **10**: 142.

80. Raz R, Stamm WE. A controlled trial of intravaginal estriol in postmenopausal women with recurrent urinary tract infections. *New Eng J Med* 1993; **329**: 753–756.

81. Cardozo LD, Benness C, Abbott D. Low dose oestrogen prophylaxis for recurrent urinary tract infections in elderly women. *Br J Obstet Gynaecol* 1998; **105**: 403–407.

82. Eriksen B. A randomised, open, parallel group-study on the preventive effect of an estradiol-releasing vaginal ring (Estring) on recurrent urinary tract infections in postmenopausal women. *Am J Obstet Gynecol* 1999; **180**: 1072–10741

83. Cardozo L, Lose G, McClish D *et al.* A systematic review of estrogens for recurrent urinary tract infections. *Int Urogynecol J* 1999; **10** (suppl 1): S32.

Hormone replacement therapy and osteoporosis

Juliet E Compston

4

Introduction

The role of oestrogen deficiency in the pathogenesis of menopausal bone loss is well established and hormone replacement therapy (HRT) has been widely used for the prevention and treatment of osteoporosis in postmenopausal women. Although prevention of postmenopausal bone loss by HRT has been convincingly demonstrated at a number of skeletal sites, evidence supporting its anti-fracture efficacy is derived almost wholly from observational studies, which are likely to overestimate any benefits and may even generate spurious effects. Over the past decade a number of non-hormonal options have become available for the prevention of osteoporotic fractures in postmenopausal women; for some of these there is robust evidence of anti-fracture efficacy from adequately powered, randomized, controlled trials. The place of HRT as the 'gold-standard' treatment for osteoporosis is thus now challenged as evidence for its effectiveness has come under greater scrutiny and uncertainties about long-term effects on coronary heart disease have emerged.

The pathophysiology of postmenopausal osteoporosis

Effects of oestrogen on bone cells

Knowledge of oestrogen signalling pathways has advanced rapidly in recent years and has facilitated the development of selective oestrogen receptor modulators, discussed elsewhere in this book. The precise mechanisms by which oestrogen exerts its beneficial effects on bone remain, however, to be clearly defined; these effects extend throughout most of the lifespan of women and probably also of men. Oestrogen-induced effects on the skeleton may be exerted via either genomic or non-genomic actions; the importance of the latter is increasingly recognized in the mediation of rapid responses to the hormone by both osteoblasts and osteoclasts.[1,2]

Oestrogen receptors belong to a family of steroid hormone receptors which includes glucocorticoid, androgen, progesterone, and mineralocorticoid receptors. At least two main subtypes of the oestrogen receptor (ER) exist, namely, ERα and β.[3] Several isoforms of ERβ and at least two of ERα, created by alternative splicing or alternative initiation of translation, have also been demonstrated, mainly at mRNA level. Both receptor subtypes have been reported in human bone; their distribution appears to be overlapping but not identical and recent evidence suggests that ERα is predominant in cortical bone

whereas ERβ is the main form in cancellous bone. Oestrogen receptors have been described on all the main cell types of bone, namely, osteoclasts,[4,5] osteoblasts,[6,7] and osteocytes.[8]

Oestrogen has effects on the production of a number of cytokines and growth factors involved in the regulation of bone remodelling (*Table 4.1*). The bone-preserving effect of oestrogen is mediated predominantly through effects on osteoclast number and activity, the latter encompassing both resorptive activity and lifespan of the cell. Oestrogen deficiency in postmenopausal women is associated with increased production of interleukin-1 (IL-1), tumour necrosis factor α (TNFα), and granulocyte-macrophage colony stimulating factor (GM-CSF),[9–11] cytokines that increase osteoclastogenesis and in the case of IL-1 and TNFα also increase osteoclastic activity. Oestrogen also inhibits the production of interleukin-6 (IL-6)[12] and, more recently, has been shown to stimulate the production of osteoprotegerin in osteoblastic cells;[13] the latter functions as a soluble decoy receptor for the cytokine RANKL (receptor activator of NFκB ligand),[14] which is essential for osteoclastogenesis. Effects of oestrogen on osteoclast activity are also mediated via stimulation of apoptosis. Thus IL-1, IL-6, and M-CSF have all been shown to inhibit apoptosis in osteoclasts,[15] whereas transforming growth factor β (TGFβ), the

Table 4.1
Effects of oestrogen on cytokines and growth factors involved in the regulation of bone remodelling.

Cytokine/growth factor	Action	Effect of oestrogen
IL-1	Pro-resorptive	⇓
IL-6	Pro-resorptive	⇓
TNFα	Pro-resorptive	⇓
M-CSF	Pro-resorptive	⇓
PGE2	Pro-resorptive	⇓
RANKL	Pro-resorptive	⇓
IL-1 receptor antagonist	Anti-resorptive	⇑
OPG	Anti-resorptive	⇑
TGFβ	Anti-resorptive	⇑
	Increased formation	⇑
BMP-6	Increased formation	⇑
IGF	Increased formation	⇑

production of which is decreased in oestrogen-deficient states, stimulates apoptosis.[16]

Several effects of oestrogen on gene expression in osteoblasts have been reported,[17] including induction of insulin-like growth factor 1 (IGF-1), TGFβ, and bone morphogenetic protein 6 (BMP-6).[18] Increased expression of alkaline phosphatase, osteocalcin, and type I collagen have also been reported in response to oestrogen in *in vitro* systems.

Bone remodelling and mechanisms of menopausal bone loss

Bone remodelling is a surface phenomenon that serves to maintain the mechanical integrity of the skeleton and to preserve calcium homeostasis (*Fig. 4.1*). Essentially it consists of the removal by osteoclasts of a quantum of mineralized bone, followed by the formation within the cavity so formed of new bone; this is initially laid down as unmineralized bone (osteoid), which then is mineralized, both these functions being performed by osteoblasts. In the adult human skeleton these processes are coupled both in space and time, bone resorption always preceding bone formation and the amounts of bone resorbed and formed being quantitatively similar (at least in the young adult skeleton). The lifespan of each remodelling unit is believed to be around 4–7 months, most of this period being occupied by formation.[19]

At the cellular and tissue level, there are

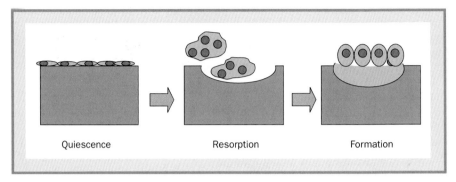

Quiescence   Resorption   Formation

Figure 4.1
Schematic diagram of bone remodelling in cancellous bone. Bone resorption by osteoclasts is followed by formation within the cavity formed of new bone by osteoblasts.

two possible mechanisms of bone loss (*Fig. 4.2*). Quantitatively the most important is an increase in activation frequency (also termed 'increased bone turnover') in which the number of remodelling units on the bone surface is increased. The second mechanism, which often coexists with increased bone turnover, is remodelling imbalance, in which the amount of bone formed within individual remodelling units is less than that resorbed, due to increased resorption, decreased formation, or a combination of the two. There is evidence from kinetic and biochemical measurements of bone turnover that increased activation frequency plays a major role in bone loss after the menopause.[20,21] In addition, histomorphometric data support a reduction in the amount of bone formed within

remodelling units, indicating decreased osteoblast activity.[22,23] There is also some evidence that oestrogen deficiency may be associated with a transient increase in osteoclastic activity,[24] resulting in increased resorption depth. This would be consistent with the observation of greater age-related disruption of cancellous bone architecture in women than in men.[25, 26]

Histomorphometric studies in postmenopausal women with osteoporosis show considerable heterogeneity in bone turnover; whether this reflects measurement variance or other factors such as regional variations or sequential or intermittent changes has not been clearly established. A more consistent finding has been a reduction in wall width, which represents the amount of bone formed within individual remodelling

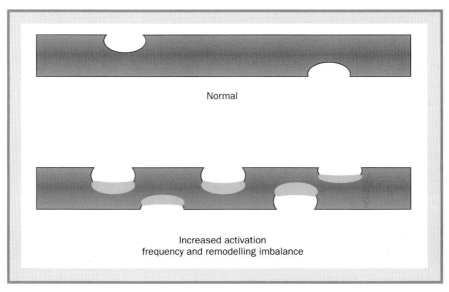

Figure 4.2
Mechanisms of menopausal bone loss. Activation frequency is increased, leading to an increase in the number of remodelling units undergoing bone resorption. Subsequent bone formation is insufficient to fill the existing resorption cavities completely.

units.[27] However, it remains unclear whether the development of postmenopausal osteoporosis reflects a distinct pathophysiological process or whether it results from physiological bone loss in those with low peak bone mass and possibly also lower levels of osteoblast activity.[28]

In premenopausal women, acute oestrogen withdrawal has dramatic effects on the skeleton. Thus treatment for a period of 6 months with gonadotrophin-releasing hormone analogues in women with endometriosis resulted in rapid disruption of cancellous architecture;[24] this is likely to have been due, at least in part, to increased resorption depth, a change that was directly demonstrated in the cortical bone of these subjects.[29]

Skeletal effects of progesterone

Relatively little is known about the skeletal effects of progesterone. Human osteoblastic cells express progesterone receptors,[7] and some progestogens used in HRT formulations, particularly 19-nortestosterone derivatives, may independently exert beneficial effects on bone mass although evidence for this is conflicting.[30–34] Thus preservation of bone mineral density in postmenopausal women treated with norethisterone was reported in metacarpal bone[30] whereas in another study[31] norgestrel therapy was associated with significant bone loss at this site in a similar cohort. In premenopausal women treated with cyclic medroxyprogesterone for menstrual disorders, increases in bone mineral density were reported.[35] There is no evidence that combined oestrogen/progestin therapy differs from unopposed oestrogen in terms of anti-fracture efficacy.[36]

Clinical aspects of postmenopausal osteoporosis

Osteoporosis is characterized by a reduction in bone mass and disruption of cancellous bone architecture, resulting in increased bone fragility and hence increased fracture risk. Fragility fractures are the only clinical manifestation of osteoporosis and most commonly occur at the hip, wrist, and spine. In women all these fractures show an age-related increase in incidence and the estimated remaining lifetime risk of developing an osteoporotic fracture in a Caucasian women at the age of 50 years has been estimated as 30–40%.[37,38] The morbidity and mortality associated with osteoporotic fractures is considerable and the estimated annual cost to the health services in the UK is around £1 billion.[39,40]

Effects of HRT on bone mineral density

Prevention of menopausal bone loss by HRT has been documented in many studies.[41–45] The beneficial effects are seen at multiple skeletal sites and can be demonstrated both in perimenopausal women and in women who are 10–20 years postmenopausal.[46] In most studies small increases in bone mineral density are seen over the first 18 months or so of treatment, typically 3–6%, followed by a plateau as the new steady state is reached. Oral, parenteral, and transdermal formulations have all been shown to be effective. There is some evidence that addition of calcium supplementation enables lower doses of oestrogen to be used.[47,48]

Effects of HRT on bone turnover and remodelling

The beneficial effects of HRT on menopausal bone loss are mediated predominantly by suppression of bone turnover. Thus biochemical markers of bone resorption and formation fall to values within the normal premenopausal range after 3–6 months of treatment[49] and several histomorphometric studies have demonstrated a significant reduction in activation frequency and bone turnover at tissue level in postmenopausal women treated with hormone replacement therapy,[50–52] generally to approximately 50% of the untreated values. The issue of whether HRT affects remodelling balance is more contentious but there is some evidence that the depth of resorption cavities, an index of osteoclastic activity, is reduced by hormone replacement therapy.[52,53] In contrast, there is no evidence that HRT, when used in conventional doses, increases bone formation at the cellular level as assessed by histomorphometric measurements of wall width.[50,52,53] Consistent with these reductions in bone turnover and osteoclastic activity, there is evidence that cancellous bone architecture is preserved by HRT although disruption occurring before therapy is not reversed.[53,54]

Effects of HRT on fracture risk

Evidence for the anti-fracture efficacy of HRT is derived almost exclusively from observational studies, which are subject to bias and likely to overestimate potential benefits because of the healthier status of those women who choose to take HRT at the menopause as compared with those who do not. Nevertheless, the majority of evidence supports the contention that HRT is effective in reducing fracture risk at the wrist, hip, and spine.[55–63] Of these studies, only a minority have been prospective[42,51,56,63] and none has been optimally designed. In this context, it is of interest that in a recent randomized, controlled trial of the effects of HRT in women with coronary heart disease no effect of HRT on clinical fractures, which were a secondary end-point, was observed.[64] The results of several ongoing large randomized, controlled trials in the UK and USA, in which effects on fragility fractures will be documented, are therefore awaited with interest.

The optimal timing and duration of HRT in the prevention of osteoporosis have not been clearly established. There is increasing evidence for attenuation of its beneficial skeletal effects after withdrawal of therapy, with respect both to bone mineral density and to fracture reduction. Thus two cross-sectional studies in postmenopausal women have provided evidence that some years after HRT is stopped benefits for bone mineral density are no longer observed[65,66] and several observational studies indicate that significant protection against hip fracture is seen only in current or recent HRT users.[59,62] (*Fig. 4.3*). Although further studies are required, in particular prospective investigations of rates of bone loss after withdrawal of therapy, these data indicate that lifelong treatment after the menopause is required to maintain optimal protection against fracture, the incidence of

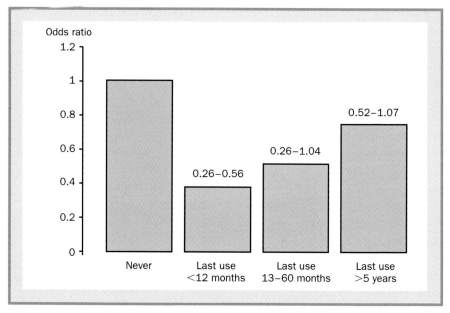

Figure 4.3
Effect of time since last use of HRT on risk of hip fracture. The greatest protection is seen in recent and current users, whereas no significant protection was observed in women who had not received HRT for 5 years or longer.[62]

which rises steeply with age and, in the case of hip fracture, reaches a peak around the age of 80 years. There has thus been a move away from long-term preventive strategies, starting at the time of the menopause, towards shorter-term intervention in older women who have a high absolute risk of fracture.

Tibolone

Tibolone, a synthetic compound, has oestrogenic, progestogenic, and androgenic

properties and is effective in the treatment of menopausal symptoms. Its effects on bone mineral density are similar to those observed with other forms of HRT;[67] however, there are at present no data on its anti-fracture efficacy.

High-dose oestrogen therapy: anabolic effects on bone

Percutaneous oestradiol therapy, which is associated with high serum oestradiol concentrations, results in greater increases in bone mineral density in postmenopausal women than do oral or transdermal formulations;[45,68,69] although early studies mainly involved co-administration of testosterone, more recently it was shown that long-term treatment of postmenopausal women with high doses of percutaneous oestradiol, in the absence of testosterone, was associated with bone mineral density values that were significantly higher than those expected in their normal premenopausal counterparts.[70] This effect is achieved, at least in part, through an increase in bone formation at the cellular level, resulting in increased wall width and improved remodelling balance.[71] The mechanisms by which oestrogens achieve osteoblastic stimulation have not been defined but may have potential implications for the development of other anabolic skeletal agents.

Monitoring of bone mineral density in patients receiving HRT

Although noncompliance with long-term HRT is common, current evidence indicates that the level of true non-response to HRT is low.[72] Although it has been argued that regular monitoring by bone densitometry may improve compliance, this cannot be justified on the basis of cost-effectiveness, and in the absence of complicating factors such as malabsorption or glucocorticoid therapy it is hard to justify such an approach.[73] It may, however, be more useful to assess bone density at the time of cessation of HRT in order to establish whether further bone-sparing therapy is required.

The positioning of HRT in the management of osteoporosis in postmenopausal women

In recent years there have been significant advances in the management of osteoporosis in postmenopausal women and the range of licensed interventions has increased considerably (*Table 4.2*).[74] For some of these agents, for example alendronate, raloxifene, and risedronate, there is robust evidence of anti-fracture efficacy from adequately powered, randomized, controlled trials; in other cases, the evidence is less robust and sometimes inconsistent. Decisions in clinical practice about which intervention to advise are affected by a number of issues, including anti-fracture efficacy for both vertebral and non-vertebral fractures, the rate of onset and offset of treatment effect, safety and tolerability, cost, and, for raloxifene and HRT, the extraskeletal risks and benefits.

Although for regulatory purposes a distinction is drawn between prevention and treatment of osteoporosis, in clinical practice this is not useful, since all currently available treatments act fundamentally in the same way, i.e. by inhibiting bone resorption. Furthermore, there is evidence that the rate of onset and offset of therapeutic effect is

Table 4.2
Summary of evidence for anti-fracture efficacy of interventions used in the prevention of osteoporotic fractures in postmenopausal women

	Spine	Non-vertebral	Hip
HRT	+	+	+[*]
Raloxifene	+	−	−
Alendronate	+	+	+
Cyclic etidronate	+[†]	+[*]	+[*]
Risedronate	+	+	+
Calcitonin	+	−	+[*]
Calcitriol	+	+	−
Vitamin D + calcium	−	+	+[†]

[*]Evidence based on observational data.
[†]Insufficiently powered clinical trials.
[‡]Reduction in hip fracture shown only in elderly living in sheltered accommodation.

Source: Reprinted from Compston JE. Prevention of osteoporotic fractures in post-menopausal women. Bailliere's Best Practice Res Clin Endocrinol Metab, 2000; **14**(2): 251–264, by permission of the publisher Bailliere Tindall.

relatively rapid for many of these agents, significant reductions in vertebral fracture being demonstrated after as little as 1 year's treatment in postmenopausal women with established osteoporosis.[75,76] It is therefore more logical to consider the indication for treatment as prevention of osteoporotic fracture, whether or not a fracture has already occurred, particularly in view of the strengthening rationale for targeting high-risk women for intervention rather than implementing long-term preventive strategies in those with low absolute risk of fracture.

The positioning of HRT in the management of postmenopausal women with osteoporosis has thus changed, as a result of both the emergence of other interventions and the move away from prevention of bone loss in perimenopausal women whose absolute risk of fracture is low. Although HRT remains the treatment of choice for osteoporosis in perimenopausal women with active menopausal symptoms who have a high absolute risk of fracture, such individuals are relatively rare, the majority of high-risk women being over the age of 65 years. Many women in this age group, in whom the frequency of unwanted side-effects of HRT is relatively high, prefer a non-hormonal option such as a bisphosphonate; furthermore, in the very elderly, in whom hip fracture is the major concern, the stronger evidence of anti-fracture efficacy of the bisphosphonates and, in institutionalized subjects, combined calcium and vitamin D therapy make these the most appropriate choice.

Conclusions

Oestrogen has important effects on skeletal health throughout childhood, adolescence, and adult life. In particular, the loss of oestrogen at the menopause results in accelerated bone loss and is a major pathogenetic factor in postmenopausal osteoporosis. Although it is well documented that oestrogen replacement at the menopause prevents bone loss, evidence for anti-fracture efficacy is based mainly on observational studies and is less robust than that now available for several other interventions, including alendronate, raloxifene, and risedronate.

The mechanisms by which oestrogen affects bone remodelling remain to be fully elucidated but the predominant effect appears to be on osteoclastic activity and bone turnover, although high doses of oestrogen increase bone formation and thus have an anabolic effect. These effects are mediated by both genomic and non-genomic signalling and involve the interdependent actions of a number of cytokines, growth factors, and other mediators.

References

1. Brubaker KD, Gay CV. Evidence for plasma membrane-mediated effects of estrogen. *Calcif Tissue Int* 1999; **64**: 459–462.

2. Endoh H, Saski H, Maruyama K *et al.* Rapid activation of MAP kinase by estrogen in the bone cell line. *Biochem Biophys Res Commun* 1997; **235**: 99–102.

3. Kuiper GGJM, van den Bemd GJC, van Leeuwen JPTM. Estrogen receptor and the SERM concept. *J Endocrinol Invest* 1999; **22**: 594–603.

4. Pensler JM, Langman CB, Radosevitch JA *et al.* Sex steroid hormone receptors in normal and dysplastic bone disorders in children. *J Bone Miner Res* 1990; **5**: 493–498.

5. Hoyland JA, Mee AP, Baird P *et al.* Demonstration of estrogen receptor mRNA in bone using in situ reverse transcriptase polymerase chain reaction. *Bone* 1997; **20**: 87–92.

6. Eriksen EF, Colvard DS, Berg NJ *et al.* Evidence of estrogen receptors in normal human osteoblast-like cells. *Science* 1988; **241**: 84–86.

7. Komm BS, Terpening CM, Benz DJ *et al.* Estrogenic binding, receptor mRNA and biologic response in osteoblast-like osteosarcoma cells. *Science* 1988; **241**: 81–83.

8. Braidman IP, Davenport LK, Carter DH *et al.* Preliminary in situ identification of estrogen target cells in bone. *J Bone Miner Res* 1995; **10**: 74–80.

9. Pacifici R, Brown C, Puscheck E *et al.* Effect of surgical menopause and estrogen replacement on cytokine release from human blood mononuclear cells. *Proc Natl Acad Sci USA* 1991; **88**: 5134–5138.

10. Pacifici R, Vannice JL, Rifas L et al. Monocytic secretion of interleukin-1 receptor antagonist in normal and osteoporotic women: effect of menopause and estrogen/progesterone therapy. *J Clin Endocrinol Metab* 1993; 77: 1135–1141.

11. Ralston SH, Russell RGG, Gowen M. Estrogen inhibits release of tumor necrosis factor from peripheral blood mononuclear cells in postmenopausal women. *J Bone Miner Res* 1990; 5: 983–988.

12. Pottratz ST, Bellido T, Mocharla H et al. 17beta-estradiol inhibits expression of human interleukin-6 promoter-reporter constructs by a receptor-dependent mechanism. *J Clin Invest* 1994; 93: 944–950.

13. Hofbauer LC, Khosla S, Dunstan CR et al. Estrogen stimulates gene expression and protein production of osteoprotegerin in human osteoblastic cells. *Endocrinology* 1999; 140: 4367–4370.

14. Kong Y-Y, Yoshida H, Sarosi I et al. OPGL is a key regulator of osteoclastogenesis, lymphocyte development and lymph-node organogenesis. *Nature* 1999; 397: 315–323.

15. Hughes DE, Boyce BF. Apoptosis in bone physiology and disease. *J Clin Pathol* 1997; 50: 132–137.

16. Hughes DE, Wright KR, Mundy GR et al. TGF beta 1 induces osteoclast apoptosis in vitro. *J Bone Miner Res* 1994; 9: S71.

17. Oursler MJ. Estrogen regulation of gene expression in osteoblasts and osteoclasts. *Crit Rev Eukaryotic Gene Expr* 1998; 8: 125-140.

18. Rickard DJ, Hofbauer LC, Bonde SK et al. Bone morphogenetic protein-6 production in human osteoblastic cell lines—selective regulation by estrogen. *J Clin Invest* 1998; 101: 413–422.

19. Parfitt AM. Osteonal and hemi-osteonal remodeling: the spatial and temporal framework for signal traffic in adult human bone. *J Cell Biochem* 1994; 55: 273–286.

20. Heaney RP, Recker RR, Saville PD. Menopausal changes in bone remodelling. *J Lab Clin Med* 1978; 92: 964–970.

21. Uebelhart D, Schlemmer A, Johansen JS et al. Effect of menopause and hormone replacement therapy on the urinary excretion of pyridinium cross-links. *J Clin Endocrinol Metab* 1991; 72: 367–373.

22. Lips P, Courpron P, Meunier PJ. Mean wall thickness of trabecular bone packets in the human iliac crest: changes with age. *Calcif Tissue Int* 1978; 26: 13–17.

23. Vedi S, Compston JE, Webb A et al. Histomorphometric analysis of dynamic parameters of trabecular bone formation in the iliac crest of normal British subjects. *Metab Bone Dis Rel Res* 1983; 5: 69–74.

24. Compston JE, Yamaguchi K, Croucher PI et al. The effects of gonadotrophin-releasing hormone agonists on iliac crest cancellous bone structure in women with endometriosis. *Bone* 1995; 16: 261–267.

25. Compston JE, Mellish RWE, Croucher PI et al. Structural mechanisms of trabecular bone loss in man. *Bone Miner* 1989; 6: 339–350.

26. Mellish RWE, Garrahan NJ, Compston JE. Age-related changes in trabecular width and spacing in human iliac crest biopsies. *Bone Miner* 1989; 6: 331–338.

27. Eriksen EF, Hodgson SF, Eastell R et al. Cancellous bone remodeling in type I [postmenopausal] osteoporosis: quantitative assessment of rates of formation, resorption, and bone loss at tissue and cellular levels. *J Bone Miner Res* 1990; 5: 311–319.

28. Croucher PI, Garrahan NJ, Compston JE. Structural mechanisms of trabecular bone loss in primary osteoporosis: specific disease mechanism or early ageing? *Bone Miner* 1994; **25**: 111–121.

29. Bell KL, Loveridge N, Lindsay PC *et al.* Cortical remodelling following suppression of endogenous estrogen with analogs of gonadotrophin releasing hormone. *J Bone Miner Res* 1997; **12**: 1231–1240.

30. Abdalla HI, Hart DM, Lindsay R *et al.* Prevention of bone mineral loss in postmenopausal women by norethisterone. *Obstet Gynecol* 1985; **66**: 789–792.

31. Hart DM, Abdalla H, Clarke D *et al.* Preservation of bone mass in postmenopausal women during therapy with estrogen and progestogens. In: Christiansen C, Arnaud CD, Nordin BEC *et al.*, eds. *Copenhagen International Symposium.* Aalborg: Aalborg Stiftsbogtrykkeri, 1984; 697–699.

32. Selby PL, Peacock SA, Barkworth SA *et al.* Early effects of ethinyloestradiol and norethisterone treatment in postmenopausal women on bone resorption and calcium regulating hormones. *Clin Sci* 1985; **69**: 265–271.

33. Riis BJ, Christiansen C, Johansen JS *et al.* Is it possible to prevent the bone loss in young women treated with LH-RH agonists. *J Clin Endocrinol Metab* 1990; **70**: 920–924.

34. Adachi JD, Sargeant EJ, Sagle MA *et al.* A double-blind randomised controlled trial of the effects of medroxyprogesterone acetate on bone density of women taking oestrogen replacement therapy. *Br J Obstet Gynaecol* 1997; **104**: 64–70.

35. Prior JC, Vigna YM, Barr SI *et al.* Cyclic medroxyprogesterone treatment increases bone density: a controlled trial in active women with menstrual disturbances. *Am J Med* 1994; **96**: 521–530.

36. Writing Group for the PEPI Trial. Effects of hormone therapy on bone density. Results from the Postmenopausal Estrogen/Progestin Interventions (PEPI) trial. *JAMA* 1996; **276**: 1389–1396.

37. Melton III LJ, Chrischilles EA, Cooper C *et al.* How many women have osteoporosis. *J Bone Miner Res* 1992; 7: 1005–1010.

38. Compston JE, Cooper C, Kanis JA. Bone densitometry in clinical practice. *BMJ* 1995; **310**: 1507–1510.

39. Cooper C, Melton LJ. How large is the silent epidemic? *BMJ* 1992; **304**: 793–794.

40. Dolan P, Torgerson DJ. The cost of treating osteoporotic fractures in the United Kingdom female population. *Osteoporosis Int* 1998; **8**: 611–617.

41. Christiansen C, Christensen MS, McNair PL *et al.* Prevention of early menopausal bone loss: conducted 2-year study. *Eur J Clin Invest* 1980; **10**: 273–279.

42. Lindsay R, Hart DM, Forrest C *et al.* Prevention of spinal osteoporosis in oophorectomised women. *Lancet* 1980; ii: 1151–1153.

43. Ettinger B, Genant HK, Cann CE. Long-term estrogen replacement therapy prevents bone loss and fractures. *Ann Intern Med* 1985; **102**: 319–324.

44. Stevenson JC, Cust MP, Gangar KF *et al.* Effects of transdermal versus oral hormone replacement therapy on bone density in spine and proximal femur in postmenopausal women. *Lancet* 1990; **336**: 265–269.

45. Ryde SJS, Bowen-Simpkins K, Bowen-Simpkins P *et al.* The effect of oestradiol implants on regional and total bone mass: a

three year longitudinal study. *Clin Endocrinol* 1994; **40**: 33–38.

46. Quigley MET, Martin PL, Burnier AM *et al.* Estrogen therapy arrests bone loss in elderly women. *Am J Obstet Gynecol* 1987; **156**: 1516–1523.

47. Ettinger B, Genant HK, Cann CE. Postmenopausal bone loss is prevented by treatment with low-dosage estrogen with calcium. *Ann Intern Med* 1987; **106**: 40–45.

48. Delmas PD, Confraveux E, Garnero P *et al.* A combination of low doses of 17β-estradiol and norethisterone acetate prevents bone loss and normalises bone turnover in postmenopausal women. *Osteoporosis Int* 2000; **11**: 177–187.

49. Uebelhart D, Schlemmer A, Johansen JS *et al.* Effect of menopause and hormone replacement therapy on the urinary excretion of pyridinium cross-links. *J Clin Endocrinol Metab* 1991; **72**: 367–373.

50. Steiniche T, Hasling C, Charles P *et al.* A randomised study of the effects of estrogen/gestagen or high dose oral calcium on trabecular bone remodelling in postmenopausal osteoporosis. *Bone* 1989; **10**: 313–320.

51. Lufkin EG, Wahner HW, O'Fallon WM *et al.* Treatment of postmenopausal osteoporosis with transdermal estrogen. *Ann Intern Med* 1992; **117**: 1–9.

52. Vedi S, Skingle SJ, Compston JE. The effects of long-term hormone replacement therapy on bone remodelling in postmenopausal women. *Bone* 1996; **19**: 535–539.

53. Eriksen EF, Langdahl B, Vesterby A *et al.* Hormone replacement therapy prevents osteoclastic hyperactivity: a histomorphometric study in early

postmenopausal women. *J Bone Miner Res* 1999; **14**: 1217–1221.

54. Vedi S, Croucher Pl, Garrahan NJ *et al.* Effects of hormone replacement therapy on cancellous bone microstructure in postmenopausal women. *Bone* 1996; **19**: 69–72.

55. Hutchinson A, Polansky SM, Feinstein AR. Postmenopausal estrogens protect against fractures of the hip and distal radius: a case control study. *Lancet* 1979; **ii**: 705–709.

56. Nactigall LE, Nachtigall RH, Nachtigall RD *et al.* Estrogen replacement therapy 1: a 10-year prospective study in the relationship to osteoporosis. *Obstet Gynecol* 1979; **53**: 277–281.

57. Weiss NS, Ure CL, Ballard JH *et al.* Decreased risk of fractures of the hip and lower forearm with postmenopausal use of estrogens. *N Engl J Med* 1980; **303**: 1195–1198.

58. Paganini-Hill A, Ross RK, Gerkins VR *et al.* Menopausal estrogen therapy and hip fractures. *Ann Intern Med* 1981; **95**: 28–31.

59. Kiel DP, Felson DT, Anderson JJ *et al.* Hip fracture and the use of estrogens in postmenopausal women: the Framingham study. *N Engl J Med* 1987; **317**: 1169–1174.

60. Naessen T, Persson I, Adami H-O *et al.* Hormone replacement therapy and risk for first hip fracture. *Ann Intern Med* 1990; **113**: 95–103.

61. Cauley JA, Seeley DG, Ensrud K *et al.* Estrogen replacement therapy and fractures in older women. Study of Osteoporotic Fractures Research Group. *Ann Intern Med* 1995; **122**: 9–16.

62. Michaëlsson K, Baron JA, Farahmand BY *et al.* Hormone replacement therapy and risk of

hip fracture: population based case–control study. *BMJ* 1998; **316**: 1858–1863.

63. Komulainen MH, Kroger H, Tuppurainen MT *et al*. HRT and Vit D in prevention of non-vertebral fractures in postmenopausal women; a 5 year randomized trial. *Maturitas* 1998; **31**: 45–54.

64. Hulley S, Grady D, Bush T *et al*. Randomized trial of estrogen plus progestin for secondary prevention of coronary heart disease in postmenopausal women. *JAMA* 1998; **280**: 605–613.

65. Felson DT, Zhang Y, Hannan MT *et al*. The effect of postmenopausal estrogen therapy on bone density in elderly women. *N Engl J Med* 1993; **329**: 1141–1146.

66. Schneider DL, Barrett-Connor EL, Morton DJ. Timing of postmenopausal estrogen for optimal bone mineral density. *JAMA* 1997; **277**: 543–547.

67. Rymer J, Chapman MG, Fogelman I. Effect of tibolone on postmenopausal bone loss. *Osteoporosis Int* 1994; **4**: 314–319.

68. Savvas M, Studd JWW, Fogelman I *et al*. Skeletal effects of oral oestrogen compared with subcutaneous oestrogen and testosterone in postmenopausal women. *BMJ* 1988; **297**: 331–333.

69. Garnett T, Studd J, Watson N *et al*. A cross-sectional study of the effects of long-term percutaneous hormone replacement therapy on bone density. *Obstet Gynecol* 1991; **78**: 1002–1007.

70. Wahab M, Ballard P, Purdie DW *et al*. The long-term effects of oestradiol implantation on bone mineral density in post menopausal women who have undergone hysterectomy and bilateral oophorectomy. *Br J Obstet Gynaecol* 1997; **104**: 728–731.

71. Vedi S, Compston JE, Ballard P *et al*. Bone remodelling and structure in postmenopausal women treated with long-term, high-dose oestrogen therapy. *Osteoporosis Int* 1999; **10**: 52–58.

72. Hassager C, Jensen SB, Christiansen C. Non-responders to hormone replacement therapy for the prevention of bone loss: do they exist? *Osteoporosis Int* 1994; **4**: 36–41.

73. Compston JE. Bone densitometry and clinical decision making. *J Clin Densitometry* 1999; **2**: 5–9.

74. Writing Group for the Bone and Tooth Society of Great Britain and the Royal College of Physicians. *Osteoporosis. Clinical Guidelines for Prevention and Treatment. Update on Pharmacological Interventions and an Algorithm for Management*. London: Royal College of Physicians of London, 2000.

75. Pols HAP, Felsenberg D, Hanley DA *et al*. Multinational, placebo-controlled, randomized trial of the effects of alendronate on bone density and fracture risk in postmenopausal women with low bone mass: results of the FOSIT study. *Osteoporosis Int* 1999; **9**: 461–468.

76. Harris ST, Watts NB, Genant HK *et al*. Effects of risedronate treatment on vertebral and nonvertebral fractures in women with postmenopausal osteoporosis. A randomized controlled trial. *JAMA* 1999; **282**: 1344–1352.

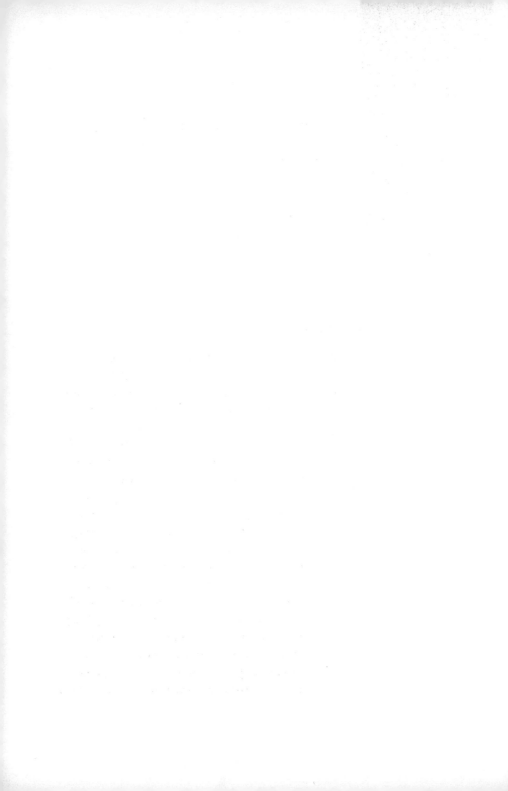

Hormone replacement therapy and heart disease

Régine Sitruk-Ware

5

Introduction

It is now well established that cardiovascular disease (CVD) represents the major cause of death in women just as in men, but at a later age. In women the incidence of CVD increases after the menopause and it has been shown that the risk of atherosclerosis increases 3–4-fold after natural menopause.[1]

Among the main recognized cardiovascular risk factors for both men and women, cigarette smoking, high cholesterol levels, hypertension, diabetes mellitus and obesity are preventable causes of coronary heart disease.[2] The fall in oestrogens following the menopause may affect several of these risk factors and it is now well established that oestrogen replacement therapy (ERT) will improve cholesterol levels, diastolic blood pressure, insulin sensitivity and some of the clotting factors.[3–6] The beneficial effects of oestrogens on the vasodilating endothelial factors, hence on vasomotor tone,[7] suggest that oestrogens may play a major role in the primary prevention of coronary heart disease in women. Better understanding of the mechanisms underlying the protective effect of sex steroids has been provided by animal studies using the monkey model[8] as well as studies of postmenopausal women, using surrogate markers of cardiovascular risk.[9,10]

There is now evidence that oestrogens will improve endothelial function and hence vascular tone,[10] however, the effect of progestogens on CVD risk is controversial. Progestins are prescribed together with oestrogens to protect the endometrium, and some of the most commonly prescribed progestins have been shown to oppose partially the beneficial effect of oestrogens on CVD risk markers.[11] However, several categories of progestins may be prescribed, and there are striking differences according to the type of molecules used.[6,12,13]

However, evidence-based medicine does not rely on surrogate markers of risk and the relationship between hormone replacement therapy (HRT) and heart disease can be demonstrated only by randomized controlled trials (RCT) with cardiovascular events as main outcomes.

Epidemiological data

Results from a large number of observational studies over the last two decades have strongly suggested that postmenopausal ERT protects against cardiovascular disease. However, this evidence is not based on randomized trials.

A number of epidemiological studies performed since the early 1980s indicate around a 50% reduction in cardiovascular morbidity and mortality in women using oestrogens after the menopause (*Table 5.1*).[14–16] However, a selection bias in the studies may account for this observation, women who take oestrogens in the long term are generally healthier than those who do not.[15,16]

The selection bias hypothesis has been reinforced by the recent results from the Heart and Estrogen/Progestin Replacement Study (HERS) research group, the first ever published RCT of HRT for secondary prevention of CVD. This study suggested that in postmenopausal women with established coronary heart disease (CHD) an HRT regimen with conjugated oestrogens (CEE) and medroxyprogesterone acetate (MPA) does not protect from further CVD.[17]

In contrast, in most observational studies of ERT and CHD, including studies conducted in women with established coronary disease,[18,19] lower cardiovascular morbidity and mortality were shown in users of ERT. Observational studies of HRT incorporating oestrogen and progestogen for primary prevention of CHD are fewer than studies of ERT,[20–24] but some show a reduction in the risk of CHD comparable to the reduction in the risk of CHD in users of HRT. The results from the observational data showing a lower risk of CHD in hormone users caused considerable debate about the ethics of randomization of women to hormone therapy, in which some subjects would receive a placebo.

Table 5.1
Key studies of combined HRT and ischaemic heart disease in postmenopausal women.

First author; year	Reference	Type of study	Treatment	Relative risk	95% CI
Falkeborn 1992	24	Cohort	E	0.69	0.54–0.86
			E + P	0.53	0.30–0.87
Psaty 1994	22	Case–control	E	0.69	0.47–1.02
			E + P	0.68	0.38–1.22
Grodstein 1996	20	Cohort	E	0.6	0.43–0.83
			E + P	0.39	0.19–0.78
Barrett-Connor 1998	16	Meta-analysis 25 studies*	E	0.7	0.65–0.75
			E + P	0.66	0.53–0.84

E = oestrogen only; E + P = oestrogen plus progestin combined HRT.
* includes the three studies above.

In her comments on the HERS study, Diana Petitti urged that caution be exercised towards observational results for CHD in users of ERT and HRT.[25] She argued that women with healthy behaviour, such as following a low-fat diet and exercising regularly, may selectively use postmenopausal hormones. These differences in behaviour may not be taken into account in the analysis of observational studies because they are not measured. Estimates of the relative risk of CHD in hormone users will then be biased towards finding a protective effect of hormone use for CHD. Barrett-Connor[26] demonstrated such a prevention bias. In two different randomized trials of drugs to prevent CHD, the subjects who faithfully took their placebo had a lower risk of CHD than subjects who were noncompliant in taking placebo.[27,28] The subjects compliant in taking placebo had 50% fewer cardiovascular events than noncompliant subjects in the Coronary Drug Project[27] and in the Beta-Blocker Heart Attack Trial.[28] A similar reduction in the relative risk of CHD was found in compliant subjects compared with noncompliant subjects taking active drug. Women included in epidemiological studies using ERT or HRT are compliant. Compliance bias is large enough to explain entirely reductions in the relative risk of CHD between users and non-users of ERT and HRT of the magnitude found in observational studies.[25] In the study of Horwitz et al[28] adjustment for multiple known predictors of coronary disease did not eliminate the decreased risk for coronary disease associated with good adherence to medication. Therefore, although the results published by several observational studies are consistent, they may reflect consistent biases.

Coronary heart disease

A recent meta-analysis by Barrett-Connor[16] of 25 studies on the relationship between HRT and CHD demonstrated a relative risk (RR) for oestrogen users of 0.7 (95% confidence interval (CI), 0.65–0.75) and 0.66 (95% CI, 0.53–0.84) for studies that assessed combined HRT. A recent epidemiological study analysing the relative risk of myocardial infarction of oestrogen/progestin users versus non-users indicated a protective effect for all therapies as compared to no treatment, even in the group using levonorgestrel, one of the most androgenic progestins used in HRT.[24]

Grodstein et al[20] reported the relationship between cardiovascular disease and HRT in 59,337 women followed for up to 16 years. Comparing the risk of major coronary

heart disease for women who did not use hormones, the relative risk was 0.6 (95% CI, 0.43–0.83) for women using oestrogens alone and 0.39 (95% CI, 0.19–0.78) for those using combined hormones. The authors found no association between stroke and use of combined hormones. For this study, conducted in the United States, the oestrogen used was mainly conjugated equine oestrogens, and the progestin most commonly used was MPA.

Although this large observational study is in accord with the previous results of Falkeborn et al[24] in Sweden and Psaty et al[22] in the United States, selection bias is possible.

The long-term randomized controlled trials in progress have been designed to eliminate such bias (*Table 5.2*).

Primary and secondary prevention trials

Several ongoing randomized trials focus on primary or secondary prevention of CHD.[17,29,30] Of the large ongoing studies, the secondary prevention trial of the HERS research group is the first published. The other trials will be completed early in the 21st century (*Table 5.2*).

Table 5.2
Key ongoing trials focusing on primary or secondary prevention of coronary heart disease.

	Steroids studied	Population	Expected results
Primary prevention			
WHI	CEE/MPA	164,000	2005
WISDOM[30]	CEE/MPA	34,000	2006
Secondary prevention			
HERS	CEE/MPA	2,763 with CHD	1998
WEST	E_2	652	?
Angiographic trials			
WELL-HART	E_2/MPA	with CHD	2001?
ERA	Placebo E/E + P	309	2000

E_2 = estradiol; E = oestrogen only; $E + P$ = oestrogen plus progestin combined HRT.

Long-term primary prevention trials

The Women's Health Initiative (WHI), in the United States, and the Women's International Study of Long Duration Oestrogen after Menopause (WISDOM), in Europe, are designed as long-term primary prevention trials and will enroll postmenopausal women without coronary disease. Long-term follow-up under treatment or placebo will help to answer questions about the presumed protective effects of HRT to prevent the occurrence of CVD and CHD.

The WHI is a large multicentre trial enrolling more than 160,000 postmenopausal women. In one subgroup of 16,500 participants the effects of HRT will be assessed. Women with a uterus will receive oestrogen plus a progestin and hysterectomized women will receive only oestrogen. The WHI will conclude around 2005 but may give earlier interim data on cardiovascular events.

The WISDOM trial is another primary prevention study. Thirty-four thousand women will be included from 12 European countries. They will receive for 10 years either conjugated equine oestrogen with or without MPA depending on uterine status, or a placebo.

Secondary prevention trials

The results of HERS do not support the beneficial effect of HRT in secondary prevention of CVD.[17] This well-designed randomized, double-blind, placebo-controlled study evaluated the role of continuous oestrogen (conjugated equine oestrogen) plus progestin (medroxyprogesterone acetate) in preventing recurrent CVD events in 2763 women with documented coronary disease.

The women were followed up for 4.1 years on average. The main objective of the study was to determine whether HRT would reduce the morbidity and mortality of cardiovascular disease. The primary outcome was the occurrence of non-fatal myocardial infarction (MI) or CHD death.

During follow-up the same number of events were recorded in both the treatment and the placebo groups. The relative hazard (RH) for a further event was 0.99 (95% CI, 0.8–1.2). There was no significant difference between groups in any of the secondary outcomes. This lack of difference in outcomes was found despite a net decrease in low density lipoprotein (LDL) and an increase in high density lipoprotein (HDL) cholesterol levels in the hormone group.

The authors concluded that they do not recommend starting HRT for secondary prevention of CHD. However, they considered it appropriate for women receiving HRT to continue, as there appeared to be a reduction of CHD in the treated group in the latter part of the trial.

Among the numerous comments published on the HERS study, Ong *et al*[31] highlighted the fact that most women included in the HERS trial were enrolled toward the end of the study period (mean 4.1 years; range 3.5–5.3 years). Since HRT was found to induce early thrombotic events and late beneficial effects (from year 3 onward), insufficient long-term follow-up of the patients recruited late in the study may have biased the results.

Although at first glance the results of HERS are disappointing, the following points are important:

1. The findings of observational research cannot be extrapolated to direct secondary prevention.
2. Although the lipid hypothesis has dominated our thinking, the mechanisms of cardiovascular disease are likely to be much more complex.
3. A negative result in secondary prevention trials does not imply such an effect in primary prevention. Postmenopausal women without previous CHD may respond to HRT differently to those with CHD.

A more recent study has challenged the assumption that HRT is cardioprotective.[32]

Duke University researchers performed an observational analysis of 1857 postmenopausal women with coronary artery disease. Nearly one-third of the women who started HRT after myocardial infarction were hospitalized with unstable angina within a year, compared with 21% of those who were already taking HRT and only 17% of those who were never on HRT. The authors concluded, as Hulley *et al*[17] previously did, that women who have heart disease should not start using HRT, but that there is no reason to suggest that women should stop using hormones if they develop heart disease while on therapy.

Angiographic trials

Angiographic trials are ongoing to compare oestrogens with and without progestins to placebo on the vessels of women with previously documented CHD. These studies may answer the question of whether HRT can slow or even reverse the accumulation of atherosclerotic plaque in the coronary arteries by providing direct evidence of anatomic changes in the arteries. The Estrogen Replacement and Atherosclerosis (ERA) study is a three-arm trial comparing a placebo group, an oestrogen-only group (CEE), and an oestrogen plus continuous progestin group

(MPA) in a total of 309 women. Angiographic information will be obtained at baseline and after three years of follow-up.* The Women's Estrogen/Progestin Lipid Lowering Hormone Atherosclerosis Regression Trial (WELL-HART) is examining the effects of oral oestradiol with or without cyclic MPA on progression of coronary stenosis.

Mechanisms of the protective effect of sex steroids on the arterial wall

From studies performed in the primate model, it is now established that sex hormones may prevent plaque formation and modulate the vasomotor response of arteries, particularly the coronary arteries. On the other hand, once the vessels are atherosclerotic, oestrogen treatment may have no effect on intimal hyperplasia or arterial remodelling in the injured artery.[33]

In the cynomolgus monkey, it has been shown that 17β-oestradiol preserves the normal endothelium-mediated dilatation of coronary arteries. However, whereas addition of cyclic or continuous MPA to oestrogens caused inhibition of vasomotor responses by 50%, natural progesterone and other non-androgenic progestins did not reverse this effect. Miyagawa *et al*[34] compared the effects of progesterone and MPA on coronary artery

---

*The results were published in August 2000. No difference was observed between placebo and active treatment in the progression of coronary atherosclerosis and clinical cardiovascular events.[40]

vasospasm, and showed that progesterone plus oestradiol protected against vasospasm but MPA plus estradiol did not. The results of the study of Williams *et al*[13] indicated that a non-androgenic progestin, nomegestrol acetate, does not diminish the beneficial effects of oestrogen on the coronary dilator response in monkeys.

Therefore, it appears that not all progestins act similarly on vasomotor tone. Different HRT combinations may affect the vascular reactivity in different ways. Current data suggest that non-androgenic molecules appear to be safer in this respect.

Unfortunately, most of the large ongoing RCTs have selected the same HRT regimen for their study design. In these circumstances we shall not get clear answers about possible beneficial effects of other treatment regimens.

Stroke and venous thromboembolism

HRT has not been shown to be consistently associated with either a reduced or increased risk of stroke of either haemorrhagic or thromboembolic origin.[16]

In recent observational studies current users of HRT have been found to be at increased risk of venous thromboembolism.[35–38] All the studies showed an increased risk of deep venous thrombosis and/or pulmonary embolism in women currently taking HRT. The relative risks were between 2.1 and 3.5 (*Table 5.3*).

The fact that risk appears to be concentrated in the first year suggests that some women, more sensitive or with predisposing factors, will develop thrombotic events with any HRT and then stop therapy, whereas the rest will remain longer-term users.

The recent results of HERS indicate that combined treatment with conjugated equine oestrogens (CEE) and MPA increased the rate of thromboembolic events in women with previous CHD, as compared with placebo (RH 2.89; 95% CI, 1.5–5.6).[17] This double-blind, randomized, placebo-controlled study confirms the results of the observational studies discussed above.

A further secondary prevention trial on that specific end-point is ongoing; the Women's Estrogen for Stroke Trial (WEST) includes 652 women and examines the effect of 17β-oestradiol in women with documented transient ischaemic attacks or stroke. The primary outcome of the trial is stroke and/or death during the 3 year study period.

Short-term trial using surrogate markers of risk

A large randomized controlled trial study on HRT and cardiovascular risk factors was published recently.[6] In the Postmenopausal Estrogen/Progestin Intervention trial[6] (the PEPI trial), 875 postmenopausal women were followed for 3 years in a randomized, double-

Table 5.3
Studies of venous thromboembolism with HRT.

First author; year	Study population	Relative risk (95% CI)
Daly 1996	VTE Case–control	3.5 (1.8–7.0)
Jick 1996	VTE Case–control	3.6 (1.6–7.8)
Grodstein 1996	PE Cohort	2.1 (1.2–3.8)
Perez-Gutthann 1997	VTE Case–control	Adjusted (Odd ratios)
	Unopposed	1.9 (1.0–3.8)
	Opposed	2.2 (1.4–3.5)
	Current use	2.1 (1.4–3.2)

VTE = venous thromboembolic events; PE = pulmonary embolism.

blind, placebo-controlled study. The three combined regimens of oestrogen and progestin induced an increase in HDL levels and a decrease in serum LDL levels. However, the increase in HDL was partially reversed in the groups where oral MPA was added to oestrogens, whereas oral micronized progesterone did not modify the oestrogen-induced rise. The results for LDL with oestrogen were not modified by the addition of a progestin, either MPA or progesterone.

However, lipid levels are only a surrogate marker of risk for CVD, accounting for only part of the presumed preventive effect of HRT. Large studies on indirect markers of risk will not give the most relevant information. This should be expected from the randomized controlled trials looking at CVD events as primary outcomes.

Conclusion

The established indications for prescribing HRT are well defined: symptom relief and consequent improvement of quality of life.

The prevention of bone fractures and CHD events remains controversial. Although several studies have demonstrated the benefits of oestrogen in decreasing postmenopausal bone loss, only a few prospective studies have shown actual prevention of fractures. For CHD the findings from observational studies are strong and consistent but several biases have been identified, the strongest of which is compliance bias. Although the secondary prevention trial of the HERS group showed no benefit for HRT in women with CHD using a given hormonal regimen, we should not extrapolate and refute the benefits of treatment as a primary prevention in normal postmenopausal women. The ongoing trials in a low-risk population should provide answers for the same hormonal regimen as in HERS. Other large trials running in Europe may indicate the effects of different hormone regimens.

The mechanisms that mediate the rapid non-genomic effects of oestrogen and the longer-term effects of oestrogen on blood vessels are not fully understood. However, rapid progress in this field may lead to more specific therapies such as oestrogens with relative selectivity for the vasculature.[39]

Until these studies are concluded, we should carefully evaluate risk factors for each individual woman and select the most appropriate therapy, favouring natural oestrogens and non-androgenic progesterone derivatives.

Acknowledgements

The author wishes to express her thanks to Nathalie Hochedez for her excellent technical assistance in preparing the manuscript.

References

1. Wittemen J, Grobbee D, Kof F *et al.* Increased risk of atherosclerosis in women after the menopause. *Br Med J* 1989; **298**: 642–644.

2. Rich-Edwards JW, Mason JE, Hennekens CH *et al.* The primary prevention of coronary heart disease in women. *N Engl J Med* 1995; **332**: 1758–1766.

3. Stevenson JC. Are changes in lipoproteins during HRT important? *Br J Obstet Gynecol* 1996; **103**(S13): 39–44.

4. Godsland IF, Gangar K, Walton C *et al.* Insulin resistance, secretion, and elimination in postmenopausal women receiving oral or transdermal hormone replacement therapy. *Metabolism* 1993; **42**: 846–853.

5. Lindoff C, Peterson F, Lecander I *et al.* Transdermal estrogen replacement therapy: beneficial effects on hemostatic risk factors for cardiovascular disease. *Maturitas* 1996; **24**: 43–50.

6. Writing group for the PEPI trial. Effects of estrogen or estrogen/progestin regimens on

heart disease risk factors in postmenopausal women: the Postmenopausal Estrogen/Progestin Interventions (PEPI) trial. *JAMA* 1995; **273**: 199–208.

7. Williams JK, Adams MR, Klopfenstein HS, Estrogen modulates responses of atherosclerotic coronary arteries. *Circulation* 1990; **81**: 1680–1687.

8. Clarkson TB, Anthony MS, Potvin Klein K. Hormone replacement therapy and coronary artery atherosclerosis: the monkey model. *Br J Obstet Gynecol* 1996; **103**(S13): 53–58.

9. Sullivan JM. Hormone replacement therapy and cardiovascular disease: the human model. *Br J Obstet Gynecol* 1996; **103**(S13): 59–67.

10. Holdright DR, Sullivan AK, Wright CA *et al.* Acute effect of estrogen replacement therapy on treadmill performance in postmenopausal women with coronary artery disease. *Eur Heart J* 1995; **16**: 1566–1570.

11. Sullivan JM, Shala BA, Miller LA *et al.* Progestin enhances vasoconstrictor responses in postmenopausal women receiving estrogen replacement therapy. *Menopause* 1995; **2**(4): 193–199.

12. Adams MR, Kaplan JR, Manuck SB *et al.* Inhibition of coronary artery atherosclerosis by 17-beta estradiol in ovariectomized monkeys. Lack of an effect of added progesterone. *Arteriosclerosis* 1990; **10**: 1051–1057.

13. Williams JK, Cline JM, Honoré EK *et al.* Coadministration of nomegestrol acetate does not diminish the beneficial effects of estradiol on coronary artery dilator responses in non human primates. *Am J Obstet Gynecol* 1998; **179**: 1288–1294.

14. Grady D, Rubin SM, Petitti DB *et al.* Hormone therapy to prevent disease and prolong life in postmenopausal women. *Ann Intern Med* 1992; **117**: 1016–1037.

15. Meade T, Berra A. Hormone replacement therapy and cardiovascular disease. *Br Med Bull* 1992; **48**(2): 276–308.

16. Barrett-Connor E. Hormone replacement therapy. *BMJ* 1998; **317**: 457–461.

17. Hulley S, Grady D, Bush T *et al.* Heart and estrogen/progestin replacement study (HERS) research group. Randomized trial of estrogen plus progestin for secondary prevention of coronary heart disease in postmenopausal women. *JAMA* 1998; **280**: 605–613.

18. Sullivan JM, Vander Zwaag R, Hughes JP *et al.* Estrogen replacement and coronary artery disease. Effect on survival in postmenopausal women. *Arch Intern Med* 1990; **150**: 2257–2562.

19. O'Brien JE, Peterson ED, Keeler GP *et al.* Relation between estrogen replacement therapy and restenosis after percutaneous coronary interventions. *J Am Coll Cardiol* 1996; **28**: 1111–1118.

20. Grodstein F, Stampfer MJ, Manson JE *et al.* Postmenopausal estrogen and progestin use and the risk of cardiovascular disease. *N Engl J Med* 1996; **353**: 453–461.

21. Rosenberg L, Palmer JR, Shapiro S. A case–control study of myocardial infarction in relation to use of estrogen supplements. *Am J Epidemiol* 1993; **137**: 54–63.

22. Psaty BM, Heckbert SR, Atkins D *et al.* The risk of myocardial infarction associated with the combined use of estrogens and progestins in postmenopausal women. *Arch Intern Med* 1994; **154**: 1333–1339.

23. Sidney S, Petitti DB, Quesenberry CP. Myocardial infarction and the use of estrogen

and estrogen–progestogen in postmenopausal women. *Ann Intern Med* 1997; **127**: 501–508.

24. Falkeborn M, Persson I, Adami HO *et al.* The risk of acute myocardial infarction after oestrogen and oestrogen–progestogen replacement. *Br J Obstet Gynaecol* 1992; **99**: 821–828.

25. Petitti DB. Hormone replacement therapy and heart disease prevention. *JAMA* 1998; **280**: 650–652.

26. Barrett-Connor E. Postmenopausal estrogen and prevention bias. *Ann Intern Med* 1991; **115**: 455–456.

27. Coronary Drug Project Research Group. Influence of adherence to treatment and the response of cholesterol on mortality in the Coronary Drug Project. *N Engl J Med* 1980; **303**: 1033–1041.

28. Horwitz RI, Viscoli CM, Berkman L *et al.* Treatment adherence and risk of death after a myocardial infarction. *Lancet* 1990; **336**: 542–545.

29. Spencer CP, Cooper AJ, Stevenson JC. Clinical trials in progress with hormone replacement therapy. *Exp Opin Invest Drugs* 1996; 5(6): 739–749.

30. Herrington DM, Potvin-Klein K. Estrogen replacement and prevention of coronary artery disease in postmenopausal women. *Menopause Management* 1998; 7: 8–19.

31. Ong PJL, Sorensen MB, Hayward CS *et al.* Hormone replacement therapy for secondary prevention of coronary disease. *JAMA* 1999; **281**: 794–795.

32. Josefson D. Women with heart disease cautioned about HRT. News on Alexander K. research presented at the Amer. Coll. Cardiol. March 7–10, 1999 (New Orleans). *BMJ* 1999; **318**: 753.

33. Geary RL, Adams MR, Benjamin ME *et al.* Conjugated equine estrogens inhibit progression of atherosclerosis but have no effect on intimal hyperplasia or arterial remodeling induced by balloon catheter injury in monkeys. *J Am Coll Cardiol* 1998; **31**: 1158–1164.

34. Miyagawa K, Rösch J, Stanczyk F *et al.* Medroxyprogesterone acetate interferes with ovarian steroid protection against coronary vasospasm. *Nature Medicine* 1997; 3(3): 324–327.

35. Perez Gutthann S, Garcia Rodriguez LA, Castellsague J *et al.* Hormone replacement therapy and risk of venous thromboembolism: population based case–control study. *BMJ* 1997; **314**: 796–800.

36. Daly E, Vessey MP, Hawkins MM *et al.* Risk of venous thromboembolism in users of hormone replacement therapy. *Lancet* 1996; **348**: 977–980.

37. Jick H, Derby LE, Myers MW *et al.* Risk of hospital admission for idiopathic venous thromboembolism among users of postmenopausal estrogens. *Lancet* 1996; **348**: 981–983.

38. Grodstein F, Strampfer MJ, Goldhaber SZ *et al.* Prospective study of exogenous hormones and risk of pulmonary embolism in women. *Lancet* 1996; **348**: 983–987.

39. Mendelsohn ME, Karas RH. The protective effects of estrogen on the cardiovascular system. *New Engl J Med* 1999; **340**(23): 1801–1811.

40. Herrington DM, Reboussin DM, Brosnihan KB *et al.* Effects of estrogen replacement in the progression of coronary-artery atherosclerosis. *N Engl J Med* 2000; **343**: 522–529.

Lipids, hormone replacement therapy and cardiovascular disease

David Crook

6

Introduction

The post-war development of analytical techniques such as ultracentrifugation and electrophoresis enabled investigators to look beyond the total lipid content of plasma and so gain insight into the complexities of intravascular lipid transport. Abnormalities of plasma lipoprotein levels were soon identified in patients with endocrine, hepatic or renal diseases, but the finding of a link with arterial diseases, such as myocardial infarction, sparked the development of detection and prevention strategies for these common but often devastating disorders. As gender differences in the plasma lipoprotein profile became apparent in the 1960s, a parallel line of research developed: the study of the effects of administered steroid hormones on lipoprotein metabolism. Oestrogens and androgens induced substantial shifts within the plasma lipoprotein profile that were in many ways consistent not only with the gender difference in the incidence of coronary heart disease (CHD) but also with emerging reports of oral-contraceptive-induced vascular disease.[1,2] Soon steroid hormones were being referred to as 'favourable' or 'unfavourable' in terms of CHD risk, solely on the basis of their metabolic effects.

The basic concept of 'biochemical risk' for arterial disease has now been validated by randomized placebo-controlled studies of statin and fibrate drugs. Protection from CHD has been demonstrated when such drugs are used to normalize plasma levels of low density lipoproteins (LDL), fasting triglycerides or high density lipoproteins (HDL).[3] As yet there is no evidence for a clinical benefit from reducing plasma levels of lipoprotein(a) (Lp(a)), but such studies are difficult to conduct in the absence of specific Lp(a)-lowering therapies.

Postmenopausal hormone replacement therapy (HRT) affects all aspects of lipoprotein metabolism (*Table 6.1*), and so there has been a strong temptation to attach clinical significance to these changes, almost to the extent of considering the plasma lipoprotein profile as a biopsy of the coronary artery. This enthusiasm is understandable, since plasma lipoprotein levels are relatively inexpensive to measure and can provide data in small trials of only a few months' duration. In contrast, studies of hard clinical end-points such as myocardial infarction cost millions of pounds and rarely take less than a decade from inception to publication.

Since plasma lipoproteins have become increasingly used to assess HRT safety, it is appropriate to audit their predictive strength in the context of steroid-induced changes. For postmenopausal HRT, the only randomized placebo-controlled trial, the Heart

Table 6.1
Plasma lipoprotein risk factors for CHD influenced by postmenopausal HRT

Fasting triglycerides
Remnant lipoproteins
Postprandial triglyceride response
LDL, especially 'small dense' LDL
ApoB
Lp(a)
LDL oxidation
HDL
HDL subfractions
ApoAI

Estrogen/progestin Replacement Study (HERS)[4] found no protection in CHD patients treated with conjugated equine oestrogens (CEE) and medroxyprogesterone acetate (MPA). Indeed, HRT users experienced a higher incidence of CHD in the early years of the study. This would conflict with the predictions of at least 50% protection, considered in part to be due to changes in plasma lipoprotein levels. In healthy women the case for a protective effect (perhaps at a lower level) remains persuasive.[5] The Women's Health Initiative,[6] due to report in 2005, should resolve this controversy.

The most obvious shortcoming to the use of plasma lipoprotein levels to assess the CHD risk of different postmenopausal therapies is that such judgements do not address the effects on other risk systems. These include the nebulous associations with endothelial function, coagulation and fibrinolysis, insulin dynamics, growth factors and so on. This is not to say that plasma lipoproteins are unimportant: only that the extent of their contribution is unknown at present. The derivation of the figure of 30% as a contribution of 'lipids' to the protection seen in observational studies of HRT users[5] is itself rather puzzling. If all the mechanisms claimed to be involved in the protective action of HRT[7] were in play then the disease would be prevented many times over. Modern concepts of plasma lipoprotein risk factors for atherosclerosis include Lp(a), postprandial lipaemia, oxidized lipoproteins, pre-β HDL and so on. These have never been measured in the context of an HRT study involving clinical end-points of CHD and so it seems premature to pin down the contribution of 'lipids' in such a way.

There is a second complication to what was once a simple story. Some steroid-induced changes in plasma lipoproteins (and other risk factors) may be cosmetic; in other words when closely scrutinized the apparent association with CHD risk may fade. Perhaps the clearest example is the increased fasting triglyceride levels induced by oral oestrogens. Women with high fasting plasma triglyceride levels are at increased risk of CHD[8] but kinetic studies of the action of oral oestrogens on triglyceride metabolism suggest that the large triglyceride-rich lipoproteins induced by therapy are

rapidly catabolized and do not become atherogenic.[9] The effect of steroid hormones on HDL, historically a major area of concern, is also being re-evaluated.[10] HRT-induced changes in lipoprotein function may be more important than changes in their plasma levels.

The effect of postmenopausal therapies on the plasma lipoprotein profile has been exhaustively reviewed over recent years[11-13] and so only new or landmark citations will be used.

HRT and plasma total cholesterol

In general, postmenopausal therapies in current use lower plasma total cholesterol levels by up to 15%. In most individuals the plasma total cholesterol level, largely determined by the level of LDL, correlates with the incidence of CHD within populations. For a hypercholesterolaemic patient, the plasma total cholesterol level can be used to monitor the effectiveness of therapy, but in the context of HRT-induced changes it is of little use. For example, small increases in the plasma total cholesterol level might be due to an effect solely on HDL, which, according to conventional concepts of risk would not be considered to be detrimental.

HRT and low density lipoproteins

Most cholesterol in human plasma is carried bound to $apoB_{100}$, contributing about 50% of the mass of each particle. The primary role of LDL is the transport of both dietary and endogenously synthesized cholesterol to peripheral tissues for use in the manufacture of cell membranes and steroid hormones. The cholesterol content of atherosclerotic plaques is largely derived from LDL, but these lipoproteins may need to be oxidatively damaged in order to be atherogenic. Peroxidation of LDL may lead to fragmentation of the protein component and the formation of reactive lipid species, impairing cellular uptake through the $apoB_{100}/E$ receptor. Oxidized LDL can also damage the endothelium and so impair vascular function. As these LDL enter the subendothelial space they may be subjected to further oxidative damage and then be complexed with other components of the arterial wall, such as Lp(a) and glycosoaminoglycans. 'Small dense' LDL may be especially atherogenic, perhaps due to their increased susceptibility to oxidative damage.

Women have lower LDL levels than men do, but this gender difference is lost when they pass through the menopause. Oral therapy with CEE or 17β-oestradiol reduces LDL cholesterol levels by 10–15%. Despite initial reports of a lack of effect, transdermal oestradiol reduces LDL cholesterol levels by about 5%[14] and indeed a vaginal ring developed as oestradiol therapy for postmenopausal women also reduces LDL levels.[15] Raloxifene lowers LDL levels by 12%, similar to the fall seen with oestrogen;[16] tibolone has no effect on levels of either LDL or apoB.[17]

Oestrogens reduce LDL levels by upregulating $apoB_{100}/E$ receptors in the liver and at other sites. Alternations in the synthesis and clearance of LDL precursors, such as very low density lipoproteins (VLDL) and intermediate density lipoproteins (IDL), may also be important. A further mechanism involves restructuring of the LDL particles. HRT-induced cholesterol depletion of some particles, forming small dense LDL, has been interpreted as an atherogenic effect.[18] However, if the atherogenicity of these lipoproteins results from their susceptibility to lipid peroxidation, then the anti-oxidant effects of oestrogen (see later) may counter any such increase in risk.

High doses of androgens and androgenic progestogens can increase LDL levels, both by inhibiting the activity of $apoB_{100}/E$ receptors and by stimulating the lipolytic conversion of VLDL and IDL to LDL. In practice, the progestogen types and doses currently used in HRT may if anything lead to further reductions in LDL cholesterol levels (*Fig. 6.1*).[19,20]

Interpretation of the potential clinical significance of these changes has been

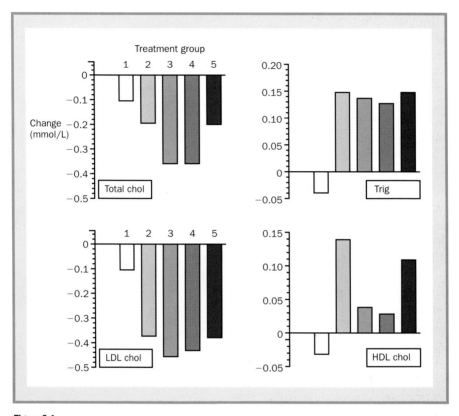

Figure 6.1

Randomized, placebo-controlled trial of the effects of oestrogen monotherapy and combined therapy on plasma lipid and lipoprotein levels. Values are mean changes over three years.[20]

Treatment groups: (1) placebo; (2) CEE 0.625 mg/day; (3) CEE 0.625 mg/day plus cyclic MPA 10 mg/day for 12 days/month; (4) CEE 0.625 mg/day plus continuous MPA 10 mg/day; (5) CEE 0.625 mg/day plus cyclic micronized progesterone, 200 mg/day for 12 days/month.

Abbreviations: CEE = conjugated equine estrogens; MPA = medroxyprogesterone acetate; Total chol = total cholesterol; HDL chol = high density lipoprotein cholesterol; LDL chol = low density lipoprotein cholesterol; Trig = fasting triglycerides.

advanced by the inclusion of women in CHD prevention trials, until recently their gender being an exclusion criterion.[21] In 1998 the results of two long-awaited trials of lipid-lowering therapy were published. Treatment of female CHD patients with pravastatin reduced the risk of subsequent disease events in one study.[22] In a study of relatively healthy individuals, the Air Force / Texas Coronary Atherosclerosis Prevention Study (AFCAPS/TexCAPS),[23] 997 women and 5608 men with low HDL levels but normal LDL levels were treated with lovastatin or placebo. LDL cholesterol levels fell by 25% and those of HDL rose by 6%. The incidence of primary cardiovascular end-points fell by 37% after five years, with both men and women being protected. Given this background, it is disappointing that the 11% fall in LDL cholesterol levels seen in HERS did not protect those women from CHD.[4]

In general, the effects of postmenopausal HRT on levels of apoB, the protein component of LDL, are rather less striking than are the effects on LDL cholesterol, consistent with structural changes within the particles. If, as is claimed, a woman's apoB level is a better predictor of her chances of developing CHD than is her LDL cholesterol level[24] then the benefits of HRT-induced reductions in LDL levels may well have been overstated.

Oestrogens protect LDL from oxidation as measured in vitro.[25] The effect in vivo is more controversial,[26] but reduced levels of antibodies to oxidized LDL have recently been shown in HRT users.[27] This finding strongly supports a clinical significance of this oestrogenic action. Oestrogen receptor mediated changes in the expression of genes for the enzymes regulating superoxide may be involved.[28] Progestogens have little effect on the ability of oestrogens to protect LDL from oxidation.[29] Tibolone prevents LDL oxidation;[30] the effect of raloxifene is unknown at present.

HRT and lipoprotein(a)

Individuals with high plasma levels of the LDL variant Lp(a) are at increased risk of CHD but only if their LDL levels are also high.[31] This lipoprotein differs from LDL by virtue of an additional peptide (apo(a)), covalently bound to the single $apoB_{100}$ molecule present in all LDL. The metabolism of Lp(a) differs from that of LDL. Lp(a) is not formed by VLDL lipolysis, nor is uptake through the $apoB_{100}/E$ receptor thought to be crucial. Apo(a) displays a high degree of structural homology with plasminogen, and may interfere with fibrinolysis. There is also a link with transforming growth factor β (TGFβ), an inhibitor of smooth muscle cell proliferation.

There may be a menopausal increase in Lp(a) levels; the evidence for an increase following oophorectomy is perhaps stronger. Most postmenopausal therapies reduce Lp(a) levels. In the PEPI study,[32] 0.625 mg/day

CEE, either alone or in combination with MPA or micronized progesterone, reduced these levels by 17–23%. Raloxifene reduces Lp(a) levels slightly (4%)[16] whereas tibolone reduces these levels by over 30%.[33] The mechanism behind these changes is unresolved. There may be an effect on hepatic apo(a) synthesis.[34] Lp(a) has many characteristics of an acute-phase protein, but the changes induced by HRT do not correlate with those in acid α-1 glycoprotein or haptoglobin.[35]

The clinical significance of such changes is difficult to predict. One attempt to retard atherosclerosis by reducing plasma Lp(a) levels with plasmapheresis failed.[36] Overall, this ability to influence Lp(a) metabolism must be regarded as an attractive side-effect of HRT, but enthusiasm must be tempered by the caution that benefit will be seen only in those women who have concomitantly high LDL levels. A recent re-analysis[37] of the HERS database has identified a subpopulation of women with elevated plasma Lp(a) levels in which HRT may have been beneficial.

HRT and triglyceride-rich lipoproteins

Oral oestrogens increase fasting plasma triglyceride levels by increasing hepatic secretion of VLDL apoB$_{100}$. CEE has more effect (about +30%) than does oral 17β oestradiol (0–15%). Transdermal or percutaneous administration of oestradiol does not increase fasting triglyceride levels, consistent with the ability of this route to avoid acutely high steroid levels in the hepatic portal vein. Indeed transdermal oestradiol often reduces fasting triglyceride levels by 10–20%,[14] consistent with the physiological effects of this hormone—premenopausal women tend to have lower fasting triglyceride levels than do age-matched men. Some of the progestogens currently used in HRT oppose the increase in fasting triglyceride levels induced by oral oestrogens, perhaps by inhibiting VLDL production.[38] The PEPI study[20] shows that the low doses of MPA and natural progesterone only weakly oppose the increase in fasting plasma triglyceride levels induced by unopposed oral CEE (*Fig. 6.1*). Raloxifene has no effect on fasting triglyceride levels;[16] tibolone reduces these levels by 25%.[17]

The increased fasting triglyceride levels seen with oral oestrogen have always conflicted with their 'favourable' image in terms of plasma lipoprotein metabolism. It has been argued that these changes are benign as they involve increased synthesis of large triglyceride-rich particles that are quickly taken up by the liver.[9] Such lipoproteins do not enter the lipolytic cascade and so resist conversion to 'remnant' lipoproteins and other atherogenic species. This defense does not exclude a detrimental effect mediated through triglyceride metabolism: the issue of secondary increases in factor VII activation needs to be addressed.[39] It would be useful to know if the striking falls in fasting triglyceride levels induced by tibolone can be linked to a fall in factor VII activation.

Fasting serum triglyceride levels are only part of the story: the postprandial response to dietary fat may be more important as a predictor of CHD events. Oral oestrogen and oestrogen/progestogen therapies improve postprandial fat clearance,[40,41] raising the possibility that the increased fasting triglyceride levels seen with some HRT formulations divert attention from a potentially beneficial effect on CHD risk.

There is an extremely rare risk of gross hypertriglyceridaemia in genetically predisposed women using oral oestrogens, similar to that seen with oral contraceptives.[42] This usually presents as severe and life-threatening pancreatitis.

HRT and high density lipoproteins

Oral therapy with CEE (0.625 mg/day) or 17β-oestradiol (1–2 mg/day) increases HDL levels by about 10%. Higher doses induce only slightly greater increases in HDL, implying that the underlying mechanisms are becoming saturated. The major mechanism involves increased hepatic synthesis of apoA1, the major structural protein of HDL.[43,44] Although oestrogens also inhibit the activity

of hepatic lipase, a key enzyme in HDL catabolism, this effect may have limited significance in vivo.[43] Transdermal oestradiol has little or no effect on HDL levels,[14] consistent with the lack of an acute effect on hepatic protein synthesis.

Progestogen can modulate oestrogen-induced increases in HDL, according to their type (C-19 versus C-21), their dose, and the balance of these factors with the type and dose of oestrogen. The route of administration of the progestogen has rather little impact. One difficulty in assessing the effects of different therapies on HDL is that clinically equivalent doses of progestogen are rarely compared. Progestogens structurally related to testosterone, such as levonorgestrel, can overcome oestrogen-induced increases in HDL levels[45] but the effect of the low doses in current use are less striking. For example, we recently evaluated an oral oestradiol/levonorgestrel intrauterine system for menopausal therapy.[46] HDL levels were unchanged by this combination, but they were similarly unchanged in a group treated with a low-dose oral oestradiol / oral levonorgestrel combination.

In the PEPI study,[20] CEE (0.625 mg/day) increased HDL cholesterol levels by 12% after six months (*Fig. 6.1*). Addition of MPA, either cyclically (10 mg/day for 12 days/month) or continuously (2.5 mg/day), blunted these increases, resulting in net increases of 3–5%. Micronized progesterone (200 mg/day for 12 days/month) was associated with less opposition to the oestrogenic effect and HDL cholesterol levels rose by about 7%. This and other controlled clinical trials show that progestogens such as levonorgestrel, norethisterone, and MPA oppose oestrogenic-induced increases in HDL, even when given at low doses in continuous regimens. This effect has been linked to increased hepatic lipase activity and the promotion of HDL catabolism. ApoA1 synthesis may also be affected. Progesterone, dydrogesterone, and related steroids have substantially less effect and maintain the oestrogenic increase in HDL levels. Raloxifene has no effect on HDL levels[16] while tibolone reduces HDL cholesterol (and apoA1) levels by 20–25%.[17]

In theory, the oestrogenic increase in plasma HDL levels is desirable. Experimental atherosclerosis is blocked in mice overexpressing the transgene for apoAI and in cholesterol-fed rabbits injected with HDL,[47] and the increased HDL levels seen in placebo-controlled trials of patients treated with gemfibrozil (a fibrate drug) have been linked to a lower incidence of CHD events.[48]

Whether the reverse is true—that HDL-reducing steroids are atherogenic—is quite a different matter. Reducing HDL levels in mice by inserting the transgene for hepatic lipase protects them from diet-induced atherosclerosis.[49] Steroid hormones may well operate through other determinants of the plasma HDL level, such as phospholipid

Table 6.2
Potential determinants of plasma HDL levels

Apolipoprotein synthesis (AI, AII, etc)
HDL assembly
LCAT
CETP
HL
LPL
Cubulin
SRB1
ABC1
Other putative receptors

transfer protein, cubulin, scavenger receptor BI (SR-B1) or the ATP-binding-cassette transporter 1 (ABC1) (*Table 6.2*). SR-B1 appears to be particularly oestrogen responsive.[50] If any of these mechanisms are in play then the clinical interpretation of HRT-induced changes in plasma HDL levels may need major reconsideration. For example, the very low plasma levels of HDL seen in hypercholesterolaemic mice overexpressing the transgene for SR-B1 are associated with almost total protection from diet-induced atherosclerosis.[51]

The current epidemiological database also suggests that the conventional views on HRT and lipoprotein metabolism may be too simplistic. Combined therapies appear (in non-randomized studies) to prevent CHD risk as strongly as does unopposed oestrogen,[52] despite the blunting of the HDL increase. In the single randomized, placebo-controlled trial of clinical events (HERS), the 10% increase in

HDL levels seen with combined therapy had no clinical effect.[4]

Hormone replacement therapy for dyslipidaemia

The ability of oral oestrogen to lower LDL levels, even against the background of a low-fat diet,[53] raises the issue of their use in hypercholesterolaemia. Following initially promising results, various double-blind comparative studies with conventional lipid-lowering drugs have now been completed. In general, these show that oral HRT on its own rarely achieves the LDL cholesterol target levels defined by national policies but, as would be predicted, has useful effects on HDL and Lp(a) which may be matched by potentially unwanted increases in fasting triglycerides.[54,55] The influence on postprandial lipaemia (see above) needs to be considered.

Combinations of HRT with statins[54,56–58] may have some advantages over statin monotherapy. Thus HRT is no substitute for conventional lipid-lowering therapy, but the combination with drugs such as statins may be useful. One complication here is that pre-existing CHD may well be the stimulus for starting lipid-lowering therapy in postmenopausal women; in such cases the adverse effects on vascular disease seen in HERS[4] need to be addressed. Statin therapy prevents CHD in women; HRT has the potential to do so.

References

1. Godsland JF, Wynn V, Crook D *et al.* Sex, plasma lipoproteins and atherosclerosis: prevailing assumptions and outstanding questions. *Am Heart J* 1987; **114**: 1467–1503.

2. Crook D, Godsland IF. Safety evaluation of modern oral contraceptives. Effects on lipoprotein and carbohydrate metabolism. *Contraception* 1998; **57**: 189–201.

3. Knopp RH. Drug treatment of lipid disorders. *N Engl J Med* 1999; **341**: 498–511.

4. Hulley S, Grady D, Bush T *et al.* Randomized trial of estrogen plus progestin for secondary prevention of coronary heart disease in postmenopausal women. *JAMA* 1998; **280**: 605–613.

5. Mendelsohn ME, Karas RH. The protective effects of estrogen on the cardiovascular system. *N Engl J Med* 1999; **340**: 1801–1811.

6. Rossouw JE, Hurd S. The Women's Health Initiative: recruitment complete—looking back and looking forward. *J Women's Health* 1999; **8**: 3–5.

7. Nasr A, Breckwoldt M. Estrogen replacement therapy and cardiovascular protection: lipid mechanisms are the tip of an iceberg. *Gynecol Endocrinol* 1998; **12**: 43–59.

8. Bengttsson C, Bjorklund C, Lapidus L *et al.* Associations of serum lipid concentrations and obesity with mortality in women: 20 year follow up of participants in prospective population study in Gothenburg, Sweden. *BMJ* 1993; **307**: 1385–1388.

9. Walsh BW, Schiff I, Rosner B *et al.* Effects of postmenopausal estrogen replacement therapy on the concentrations and metabolism of plasma lipoproteins. *N Engl J Med* 1991; **325**: 1196–1203.

10. Crook D. Tibolone and the risk of arterial disease. *J Br Menopause Soc* 1999; **S1**: 30–33.

11. Rijpkema AHM, van der Sanden AA, Ruijs AHC. Effects of postmenopausal oestrogen–progestogen replacement therapy on serum lipids and lipoproteins: a review. *Maturitas* 1990; **12**: 259–286.

12. Crook D. Effects of estrogens and progestogens on plasma lipids and lipoproteins. In: Fraser IS, Jansen RPS, Lobo RA *et al*, eds. *Estrogens and Progestogens in Clinical Practice*. London: Churchill Livingstone, 1998, 787–798.

13. Pickar JH, Thorneycroft I, Whitehead M. Effects of hormone replacement therapy on the endometrium and lipid parameters: a review of randomized clinical trials, 1985 to 1995. *Am J Obstet Gynecol* 1998; **178**: 1087–1099.

14. Crook D. Will the route of administration influence the potential cardiovascular benefits of postmenopausal hormone replacement therapy? *J Br Menopause Soc* 1999; **5**: 35–40.

15. Nash HA, Brache V, Alvarez-Sanchez F *et al*. Estradiol delivery by vaginal rings: potential for hormone replacement therapy. *Maturitas* 1997; **26**: 27–33.

16. Walsh BW, Kuller LH, Wild RA *et al*. Effects of raloxifene on serum lipids and coagulation factors in healthy postmenopausal women. *JAMA* 1998; **279**: 1445–1451.

17. Crook D. Tibolone (Livial): recent developments in the cardiovascular risk profile. *Climacteric* 1999; 2(suppl 1): 103.

18. Rajman I, Lip GY, Cramb R *et al*. Adverse change in low-density lipoprotein subfractions profile with oestrogen-only hormone replacement therapy. *QJM* 1996; **89**: 771–778.

19. Crook D, Cust MP, Gangar KF *et al*. Comparison of transdermal and oral estrogen/progestin hormone replacement therapy: effects on serum lipids and lipoproteins. *Am J Obstet Gynecol* 1992; **166**: 950–955.

20. Writing Group for the PEPI Trial. Effects of estrogen or estrogen/progestin regimens on heart disease risk factors in postmenopausal women. *JAMA* 1995; **273**: 199–208.

21. Thomas JL, Braus PA. Coronary artery disease in women. A historical perspective. *Arch Intern Med* 1998; **158**: 333–337.

22. The Long-Term Intervention with Pravastatin in Ischaemic Disease (LIPID) Study Group. Prevention of cardiovascular events and death with pravastatin in patients with coronary heart disease and a broad range of initial cholesterol levels. *N Engl J Med* 1998; **339**: 1349–1357.

23. Downs JR, Clearfield M, Weis S *et al*. Primary prevention of acute coronary events with lovastatin in men and women with average cholesterol levels: results of AFCAPS/TexCAPS. Air Force/Texas Coronary Atherosclerosis Prevention Study. *JAMA* 1998; **279**: 1615–1622.

24. Westerveld HT, van Lennep JE, van Lennep HW *et al*. Apolipoprotein B and coronary artery disease in women: a cross-sectional study in women undergoing their first coronary angiography. *Arterioscler Thromb Vasc Biol* 1998; **18**: 1101–1107.

25. McManus J, McEneny J, Young IS *et al*. The effect of various oestrogens and progestogens on the susceptibility of low density lipoproteins to oxidation *in vitro*. *Maturitas* 1996; **25**: 125–131.

26. Santanam N, Shern-Brewer R, McClatchey R *et al*. Estradiol as an antioxidant: incompatible

with its physiological concentrations and function. *J Lipid Res* 1998; **39**: 2111–2118.

27. Hoogerbrugge N, Zillikens MC, Jansen H *et al*. Estrogen replacement decreases the level of antibodies against oxidized low-density lipoprotein in postmenopausal women with coronary heart disease. *Metabolism* 1998; **47**: 675–680.

28. Arnal JF, Clamens S, Pechet C *et al*. Ethinylestradiol does not enhance the expression of nitric oxide synthase in bovine endothelial cells but increases the release of bioactive nitric oxide by inhibiting superoxide anion production. *Proc Natl Acad Sci (USA)* 1996; **93**: 4108–4113.

29. Arteaga E, Rojas A, Villaseca P *et al*. In vitro effect of estradiol, progesterone, testosterone, and of combined estradiol/progestins on low density lipoprotein (LDL) oxidation in postmenopausal women. *Menopause* 1998; **5**: 16–23.

30. Farish E, Barnes JF, O'Donoghue F. A comparison of the effects of two 'no-bleed' HRT regimens on cardiovascular risk factors. *Climacteric* 1999; **2** (suppl 1): 231.

31. Maher VMG, Brown BG. Lipoprotein(a) and coronary heart disease. *Curr Op Lipidology* 1995; **6**: 229–235.

32. Espeland MA, Marcovina SM, Miller V *et al*. Effect of postmenopausal hormone therapy on lipoprotein(a) concentration. PEPI investigators. Postmenopausal Estrogen/Progestin Interventions. *Circulation* 1998; **97**: 979–986.

33. Rymer J, Crook D, Sidhu M *et al*. Effects of tibolone on serum concentrations of lipoprotein(a) in postmenopausal women. *Acta Endocrinologica (Copenh)* 1993; **128**: 259–262.

34. Su W, Campos H, Judge H *et al*. Metabolism

of apo(a) and apoB100 of lipoprotein(a) in women: effect of postmenopausal estrogen replacement. *J Clin Endocrinol Metab* 1998; **83**: 3267–3276.

35. Tuck CH, Holleran S, Berglund L. Hormonal regulation of lipoprotein(a) levels: effects of estrogen replacement therapy on lipoprotein(a) and acute phase reactants in postmenopausal women. *Arterioscler Thromb Vasc Biol* 1997; **17**: 1822–1829.

36. Thompson GR, Maher VM, Matthews S *et al*. Familial Hypercholesterolaemia Regression Study: a randomised trial of low-density-lipoprotein apheresis. *Lancet* 1995; **345**: 811–816.

37. Shlipak MG, Simon JA, Vittinghoff E. Estrogen and progestin, lipoprotein (a), and the risk of recurrent coronary heart disease events after menopause. *JAMA* 2000; **283**: 1845–1852.

38. Wolfe BM, Huff MW. Effects of low dose progestin-only administration upon plasma triglycerides and lipoprotein metabolism in postmenopausal women. *J Clin Invest* 1993; **92**: 456–461.

39. Anonymous. Randomised comparison of oestrogen versus oestrogen plus progestogen hormone replacement therapy in women with hysterectomy. Medical Research Council's General Practice Research Framework. *BMJ* 1996; **312**: 473–478.

40. Westerveld HT, Kock LAW, van Rijn HJM *et al*. 17β-estradiol improves postprandial lipid metabolism in postmenopausal women. *J Clin Endocrinol Metab* 1995; **80**: 249–253.

41. Weintraub M, Grosskopf I, Charach G *et al*. Hormone replacement therapy enhances postprandial lipid metabolism in postmenopausal women. *Metabolism* 1999; **48**: 1193–1196.

42. Crook D. HRT and hypertriglyceridemias. In: Whitehead MI, ed. *The Prescriber's Guide to Hormone Replacement Therapy.* Carnforth (Lancs): Parthenon, 1998, 183–192.

43. Brinton EA. Oral estrogen replacement therapy in postmenopausal women selectively raises levels and production rates of lipoprotein A-I and lowers hepatic lipase activity without lowering the fractional catabolic rate. *Arterioscler Thromb Vasc Biol* 1996; **16**: 431–440.

44. Walsh BW, Li H, Sacks FM. Effects of postmenopausal hormone replacement with oral and transdermal estrogen on high density lipoprotein metabolism. *J Lipid Res* 1994; **35**: 2083–2093.

45. Hirvonen E, Malkonen M, Manninen V. Effects of different progestogens on lipoproteins during postmenopausal replacement therapy. *N Engl J Med* 1981; **304**: 560–563.

46. Crook D, Hampton N, Masters T. Randomised comparison of serum lipoprotein levels in postmenopausal women treated with oral oestradiol and either intrauterine or oral levonorgestrel (submitted for publication).

47. Luoma PV. Gene activation, apolipoprotein A-I/high density lipoprotein, atherosclerosis prevention and longevity. *Pharmacol Toxicol* 1997; **81**: 57–64.

48. Rubins HB, Robins SJ, Collins D *et al.* Gemfibrozil for the secondary prevention of coronary heart disease in men with low levels of high-density lipoprotein cholesterol. Veterans Affairs High-Density Lipoprotein Cholesterol Intervention Trial Study Group. *N Engl J Med* 1999; **341**: 410–411.

49. Busch SJ, Barnhart RL, Martin GA *et al.* Human hepatic triglyceride lipase expression reduces high density lipoprotein and aortic cholesterol in cholesterol-fed transgenic mice. *J Biol Chem* 1994; **269**: 16376–16382.

50. Landshultz KT, Pathak RK, Rigotti A *et al.* Regulation of scavenger receptor, class B, type 1, a high density lipoprotein receptor, in liver and steroidogenic tissues of the rat. *J Clin Invest* 1996; **98**: 984–995.

51. Arai T, Wang N, Bezouevski M *et al.* Decreased atherosclerosis in heterozygous low density lipoprotein receptor-deficient mice expressing the scavenger receptor BI transgene. *J Biol Chem* 1999; **274**: 2366–2371.

52. Grodstein F, Stampfer MJ, Manson JE *et al.* Postmenopausal estrogen and progestin use and the risk of cardiovascular disease. *N Engl J Med* 1996; **335**: 453–461.

53. Denke MA. Effects of continuous combined hormone-replacement therapy on lipid levels in hypercholesterolemic postmenopausal women. *Am J Med* 1995; **99**: 29–35.

54. Sbarouni E, Kyriakides ZS, Kremastinos DTh. The effect of hormone replacement therapy alone and in combination with simvastatin on plasma lipids of hypercholesterolemic postmenopausal women with coronary artery disease. *J Am Coll Cardiol* 1998; **32**: 1244–1250.

55. Darling GM, Johns JA, McCloud PI *et al.* Estrogen and progestin compared with simvastatin for hypercholesterolemia in postmenopausal women. *N Engl J Med* 1997; **337**: 595–601.

56. Davidson MH, Testolin LM, Maki KC *et al.* A comparison of estrogen replacement, pravastatin, and combined treatment for the management of hypercholesterolemia in postmenopausal women. *Arch Intern Med* 1997; **157**: 1186–1192.

57. Ohta H, Komukai S, Sugimoto I *et al.* Effect of a HMG-CoA reductase inhibitor combined with hormone replacement therapy on lipid metabolism in Japanese women with hypoestrogenic lipidemia: a multicenter double-blind controlled prospective study. *Maturitas* 1998; **29**: 163–171.

58. Koh KK, Cardillo C, Bui MN *et al.* Vascular effects of estrogen and cholesterol-lowering therapies in hypercholesterolemic postmenopausal women. *Circulation* 1999; **99**: 354–360.

Hormone replacement therapy and vascular flow

Michael S Marsh

7

Introduction

The majority of women seek hormone replacement therapy (HRT) for control of climacteric symptoms but many women are now considering using HRT for its long-term effects. It is clear that HRT reduces the rate of osteoporotic fracture but the possible importance of the effects of HRT on cardiovascular disease are less well understood by both physicians and patients. A recent survey[1] of 337 perimenopausal and postmenopausal women (mean age 50 years) who had graduated from Stanford University in the late 1960s examined their expectations of future health. When asked about their risk of developing coronary artery disease, three-quarters of the women thought that their risk by age 70 was less than 1%. Their true lifetime risk of developing coronary artery disease is as high as 50%.

Cardiovascular disease is the commonest cause of mortality in the Western world. It is responsible for 50% of all female deaths. There is now considerable evidence that oestrogen replacement therapy (ERT) users have almost half the incidence of coronary heart disease (CHD) than non-users[2–4] and, although health behaviour and compliance differ between users and non-users of ERT, it is likely that the difference in CHD incidence is due to an effect of oestrogen.

In women who have not had a hysterectomy HRT is usually administered in combination with progestogen to prevent endometrial carcinoma.[5] Studies of the effects of progestogens on risk markers for cardiovascular disease suggest that progestogens oppose some of the cardiovascular benefits of oestrogens on risk markers while enhancing others. It is at present not clear if the progestogens commonly used in HRT regimens will reduce or abolish the likely beneficial impact of oestrogen replacement on the incidence of CHD in postmenopausal women.

Synthetic progestogens bind to progesterone receptors but exhibit differing degrees of androgenicity. In general, C-21 steroids derived from progesterone have a high affinity for progesterone receptors and have minimal androgenic activity, whereas progestogens derived from testosterone and 19-nortestosterone have more androgenic activity. It is likely that the cardiovascular effects of different progestogens are in part related to their differing androgenicity.

Progestogens may be added to oestrogen to protect the endometrium either sequentially or every day in a continuous combined regimen. The time course of progestogen used in an HRT regimen may be as important as the type of progestogen. The progestogen-free days in a cycle of sequential HRT may be time when oestrogenic effects on cardiovascular risk markers predominate. Such periods may not occur in continuous combined regimens of HRT.

Evidence for the effect of oestrogen replacement therapy on CHD risk

Although two hospital case–control studies have found no effect of oestrogen use on heart disease[6,7] and one found an increased risk,[8] most case–control studies have shown a reduced risk in ERT users. Two of the studies showing no beneficial effect were limited to women under 50 years[6] and 46 years of age.[8] It is unlikely that these findings can be generalized to the whole postmenopausal population. The relative risks from community-based case–control studies range from 0.3 to 0.9.[9–11] In only one[11] was the relationship statistically significant.

Prospective studies of ERT use also support a beneficial effect. Bush and co-workers[3] reported an age-adjusted relative risk of myocardial infarction (MI) among users compared with non-users of 0.34 (CI 0.12–0.81), which was little affected by risk factor adjustment. The Nurses Health Study[12] reported a relative risk of MI for ERT ever users compared with never users of 0.5 (CI 0.3–0.8). The relative risk in current *versus* never users was 0.3 (CI 0.2–0.6). The relative risk in past users *versus* never users was 0.7 but was not significant, suggesting that the effects of oestrogen HRT may disappear after treatment is withdrawn. Adjustment for risk factors did not substantially change the risk estimates. Further follow-up of these women for up to 10 years[13] and 16 years[14] showed similar results. Studies that compared the extent of coronary artery occlusion at arteriography between ERT users and non-users have shown decreased stenosis in ERT users.[15-17] (*See Fig. 7.1.*)

There is evidence that oestrogen-only

hormone replacement may be useful in the secondary prevention of coronary heart disease. Sullivan and co-workers[18] retrospectively followed up for 10 years 2268 women aged over 55 years who had undergone angiography. Subjects were divided into those with less than 70% coronary artery stenosis (*n* = 644), those with more than 70% (*n* = 1178), and those without stenosis (*n* = 446). The end-point was mortality from all causes. At 10 years the survival for HRT users and never users was 97% and 60%, respectively (*P* = 0.007), in the group with the

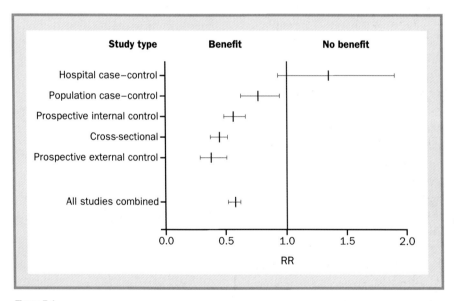

Figure 7.1
*Relative risk and 95% confidence interval estimates of coronary disease associated with ERT use. (Modified with permission from Stampfer MJ, Colditz GA. Estrogen replacement therapy and coronary heart disease: a quantitative assessment of the epidemiological evidence. Preventive Medicine 1991; **20**: 47–63.)*

most severe stenosis. Significant differences were also seen in the women with less severe stenosis. However, the authors acknowledged that there were problems with the study, e.g. never users of HRT were older and smoked more than users.

Evidence for the effect of oestrogen and progestogen replacement therapy on CHD risk

In most trials of the effects of HRT discussed above, progestogen use was infrequent. However, in two prospective studies progestogen use was more common. Hunt and co-workers[19] studied mortality secondary to a variety of causes in 4544 postmenopausal women attending specialist menopause clinics and compared them with those expected for the general female population of England and Wales, matched for age. HRT takers had all used HRT for at least 1 year. Forty-three per cent of the treatments incorporated a progestogen. Recruitment started in 1978 and mortality was assessed in 1984 and 1988. The relative risk of mortality from ischaemic heart disease at the first follow-up was 0.48 (CI 0.29–0.74), and 0.41 (CI 0.24–0.84) at the second. It is very likely that the menopause clinic attenders in this study were more health aware and health compliant than the general population.

Falkeborn and co-workers[20] followed up 23,174 women for an average of 5.8 years. They determined HRT use by questionnaire and from pharmacy records. The median age at entry was 53.9 years. The relative risk of admission to hospital with first MI for HRT ever users compared with never users was 0.81 (CI 0.71–0.92). Of these women 11% had received progestogens. In the subgroup of women who were less than 60 years of age and who received oral oestradiol/levonorgestrel HRT the relative risk was 0.53 (CI 0.3–0.87).

In the recent report from the Nurses Health Study Grodstein and co-workers[14] specifically addressed the question of CHD and oestrogen/progestogen use in a 16 year follow-up of 59,337 women who were 30–55 years of age at baseline. From 1976 to 1992 there were 770 cases of myocardial infarction or death from coronary artery disease. These authors reported less risk of major coronary heart disease among women who took oestrogen with progestogen (multivariate adjusted relative risk 0.39; 95% CI 0.19–0.78) or oestrogen alone (relative risk 0.60; 95%, 0.43–0.83), as compared with women who did not use hormones. It is likely that the large majority of women using oestrogen–progestogen therapy in this study were using a sequential regimen.

The results of the first randomized, controlled trial on hormone replacement therapy in the secondary prevention of cardiovascular disease were published recently.[21] A total of 2763 postmenopausal women with established coronary artery disease (mean age 67 years) were randomized to receive either placebo or continuous combined conjugated equine estrogens (CEE) 0.625 mg/day plus medroxyprogesterone acetate (MPA) 2.5 mg/day. The average follow-up was 4.1 years and the primary outcome was non-fatal MI or any other CHD-related death. The incidence of CHD events with hormone replacement therapy or placebo during the 5 year observation period was not different. The lack of a clear secondary prevention of coronary artery disease with hormone replacement therapy occurred despite a net 11% lower low density lipoprotein (LDL) level and 10% higher high density lipoprotein (HDL) level in the hormone group compared with the placebo group.

Mechanisms for the effect of HRT on CHD

The mechanisms by which ERT reduces the risk of myocardial infarction are not completely understood but the effect is likely to be partly via an effect on atherosclerosis. Postmenopausal women who take HRT appear to have less atherosclerosis than those who do not. In a recent study[22] of the prevalence and the extent of carotid atherosclerosis measured by ultrasound, 2588 postmenopausal women participated in a population health survey. Women with late menopause and women who had ever used postmenopausal oestrogens had significantly less atherosclerosis than women with early menopause and those who had never used oestrogen. It is uncertain whether such differences owe to the effect of oestrogens on lipids and lipoproteins (Chapter 6) and insulin metabolism (Chapter 8) or to direct vascular effects.

Direct vascular effects of HRT

Oestrogens and blood pressure

Oral natural oestrogens do not appear to cause a mean rise in blood pressure (BP)[23,24] although in a small number of women (less than 2%) the BP will rise at the beginning of therapy.[25] The effect to increase BP may be mediated via renin substrate, which may be less affected by low-dose oral or transdermal therapy than by high-dose oral therapy.

A 3 year prospective randomized double-blind placebo-controlled study examined the effect of HRT on blood pressure in 875 postmenopausal women over 3 years.[26] Subjects were treated with CEE 0.625 mg/day combined with either MPA or micronized progesterone given sequentially or continuously. Mean systolic blood pressure rose in all groups, including those assigned to placebo. There were no significant differences in the change in systolic blood pressure between women receiving HRT or those receiving placebo. Mean diastolic blood pressure did not change. Hormone replacement therapy is not obviously contra-indicated in hypertensive women, although careful supervision is needed.

Oestrogens and the vasculature

It seems clear that oestrogens have direct effects on blood flow and arterial tone. Effects such as reduced resistance to blood flow and increased vessel elasticity may lower MI risk either by reducing the likelihood of acute coronary artery vasospasm or by lessening atheroma formation.

Oestrogen receptor associated protein has been found in the arterial wall muscularis.[27] and oestrogens are known to cause release of vasoactive substances such as prostacyclin[28] and nitric oxide.[29] Oestradiol has an ionotropic effect in animals, increasing cardiac output and causing systemic vasodilatation.[30] Acute administration of oestrogen at a dose higher than those used in HRT appears to reduce myocardial ischaemia in women with coronary artery disease.[31]

In a series of studies using Doppler ultrasound to measure parameters of flow it has been demonstrated that oestrogens administered to postmenopausal women reduce the pulsatility index (PI), a measure of downstream impedance to flow, in the uterine[32,33] and internal carotid arteries.[34] The

effect on the internal carotid artery occurs with oestrogens delivered either transdermally[34] or orally.[35] (*See Fig. 7.2.*)

A recent study using a different methodology has confirmed these effects on parameters of blood flow in other vessels. In a double-blind study of the vascular reactivity of the brachial artery, Al-Khalili and co-workers[36] randomized 11 postmenopausal women to receive 2.5 or 5 mg of conjugated oestrogen or placebo intravenously. The reactive hyperemia of the brachial artery was studied before and 30 minutes after administration. The flow-mediated vasodilation at baseline before drug administration was 1.8%, after an average 400% increase in local blood flow. Conjugated oestrogen at a dose of 2.5 mg caused an increase in flow-mediated vasodilation from 1.8% at baseline to 5.4% after infusion ($P < 0.05$ versus placebo), whereas 5 mg caused an increase from 1.9% at baseline to 7.0% ($P < 0.05$ versus placebo).

It appears that the short-term effects of oestrogens on vascular tone are not related to changes in lipids and lipoproteins. In a recent double-blind, double-dummy placebo-controlled 6 month study[37] 45 apparently healthy Caucasian non-obese non-smoking hysterectomized postmenopausal women were recruited who had not received HRT for at least 3 months. They were randomized to receive either transdermal 17β-oestradiol 50 μg/day (Estraderm TTS 50 patches, Ciba-

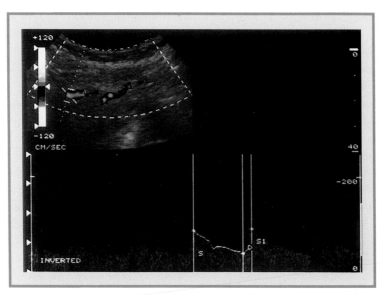

Figure 7.2
Ultrasound screen view during measurement of carotid artery pulsatility index. Image at the top left shows identification of internal and external carotid arteries (shown in purple) by colour flow mapping. Doppler ultrasound waveform is shown below.

Geigy, Horsham, UK) and placebo tablets, or conjugated equine oestrogens 0.625 mg/day (Premarin, Wyeth-Ayerst, Maidenhead, UK) and placebo transdermal patches, or placebo versions of both oestrogens. Internal carotid artery PI fell in all three groups but significantly more so than placebo in those women receiving oral or transdermal therapy. Lipids and lipoproteins were also studied. Transdermal and oral therapy had markedly different effects on serum triglcyerides — transdermal therapy lowering triglycerides by 11–14% whereas oral therapy increased

triglycerides by 27–40%. The two forms of oestrogen therapy also differed in their effects on serum LDL and HDL cholesterol. Serum LDL cholesterol was not altered by transdermal therapy but was reduced by approximately 15% by oral therapy. Oral therapy increased serum HDL by 14–21%, of which the greater increase was seen in the HDL2 subfraction. There was a small but non-significant fall in serum HDL with transdermal therapy, accounted for by a fall in HDL3 and no change or a small increase in HDL2. Most importantly, neither the direction nor magnitude of the changes in PI were related to any of the changes in lipids or lipoproteins.

The mechanism for the effect of oestrogens on the vasculature may be via endothelium-dependent or endothelium-independent mechanisms. An endothelium-dependent effect is supported by the findings of Williams and co-workers.[38] Oophorectomized cynomolgus monkeys fed with an atherogenic diet showed a paradoxical constriction of coronary arteries in response to acetylcholine compared with the usual endothelium-dependent coronary vasodilatation seen in animals on a normal diet. However, oophorectomized monkeys fed with an atherogenic diet given oestrogens showed the normal vasodilatory response to acetylcholine, suggesting an oestrogen effect on endothelial function.

Similar effects have now been shown in humans. Collins *et al*[39] studied responses of coronary arteries to acetylcholine in women with coronary artery disease. There was a paradoxical constriction of the diseased arteries to acetylcholine but this response normalized to a dilatation response following intracoronary infusion of 17β-oestradiol. This dilatation was accompanied by a significant increase in coronary flow.

There is some evidence that oestrogens act independently of the endothelium, possibly by acting as a calcium antagonist. 17β-oestradiol has also been shown to relax rabbit coronary arteries constricted by endothelin-1, and it has also been found to inhibit inward calcium currents and reduce intracellular free calcium in isolated cardiac monocytes.[40,41] The arterial vasodilatation produced by the addition of 17β-oestradiol to isolated rabbit coronary rings is still seen when the vascular endothelium is removed[42] and the vasoconstriction produced by increasing the calcium concentration is antagonized in a dose-dependent manner by 17β-oestradiol.[40] However, a recent[43] double-blind placebo-controlled crossover trial of vascular reactivity in the brachial artery in 13 postmenopausal women demonstrated an endothelium-dependent effect of oestrogens but failed to show an endothelium-independent effect. Women aged 44–69 years (mean 55 years) were randomized to receive placebo, oral oestradiol 1 mg/day, or oral oestradiol 2 mg/day for 9 weeks. High-resolution ultrasonography was used to measure vascular reactivity in the brachial artery. Endothelium-dependent vasodilatation was determined by measuring the change in brachial artery diameter during increases in flow induced by reactive hyperemia. Endothelium-independent vasodilation was measured after sublingual nitroglycerin was administered. Flow-mediated, endothelium-dependent vasodilation of the brachial artery was greater when patients received oestradiol (13.5% and 11.6% for 1 mg and 2 mg doses, respectively) than when patients received placebo (6.8%;

$P < 0.05$ for each dose compared with placebo). In contrast, oestrogen administration had no effect on endothelium-independent vasodilation as assessed by sublingual nitroglycerin.

Vascular function may be affected by changes in angiotensin II and kinins mediated by angiotensin-converting enzyme (ACE). Elevation of serum ACE is associated with an increased risk of coronary heart disease.[43] Proudler *et al*[44] demonstrated that ACE activity fell by 20% in 28 women treated with continuous combined oestradiol and norethisterone therapy over 6 months, but remained unchanged in a control group of 16 untreated women.

The effect of progestogens on the vasculature

It appears that progestogens can reverse the effects of oestrogens on vascular flow, although some studies do not report such an effect. Differences in study design and methods of assessing parameters of vascular flow may explain differences between studies.

In a study of sequential HRT incorporating norethisterone[45] it was found that the uterine artery PI was higher (by about 13%) during the oestrogen plus progestogen phase than during the oestrogen-only phase in both cycles, but still remained lower (by approximately 33%) than before treatment. In contrast to studies of oestrogen use alone on

PI a recent study[46] of carotid artery blood flow failed to demonstrate an overall effect on PI with oestrogen and progestogen HRT, suggesting that progestogens obtund the effect of oestrogens. Fifty healthy women 6 months postmenopausal were randomized to receive either placebo or 2 mg oestradiol (E2) for 12 days, to which was added 1 mg norethisterone acetate for 10 days, followed by 1 mg E2 for 6 days, cyclically over 6 months. The placebo group took placebo for the first 3 months and active treatment for the last 3 months. Pulsatility index did not decrease significantly in the common internal or external carotid arteries during 6 months of HRT in this study.

In contrast, the study of Penotti and co-workers[47] reported a rise in PI with time in women taking placebo but no change in PI in women using a sequential therapy in which progestogen was used for 12 days every 2 months. Doppler ultrasonography was used to measure PI of the internal carotid and middle cerebral arteries of 23 women who received continuous transdermal oestradiol replacement therapy (50 µg/day) to which was added medroxyprogesterone acetate 10 mg/day for 12 days every second month for 6 months in a 12 month crossover design. In the first 6 months the PI rose in the patients on placebo but did not change in those receiving HRT. After the crossover the PI dropped to values similar to those at baseline in the patients who resumed HRT and increased in those who stopped active therapy. The increase in PI in the placebo group over a relatively short time has not been reported in other studies.

Another study[48] comparing effects of oral and transdermal HRT on carotid and uterine artery vascular impedance also found no major effect of progestogen. Sixty-three postmenopausal women were randomized to 12 months' treatment with oral or transdermal sequential combined HRT. In 30 women, Doppler measurements were taken in the oestrogen–progestin combined phase. The carotid and uterine artery PI decreased with both regimens. Addition of norethisterone acetate did not appear to counteract oestrogen-induced falls in carotid and uterine PI in either group.

No effect of progestogen was seen in a recent prospective randomized operator-blinded controlled study of 68 women who had undergone surgical menopause.[49] Women were randomized to no treatment, oral oestrogen, continuous combined oestrogen and progestogen, or transdermal oestrogen. The PI of the brachial, dorsalis pedis, popliteal, and radial arteries were measured before treatment and after 2 and 6 months of treatment. There was a significant reduction in the PI in at least one of the four arteries after 2 months of HRT in all the treatment groups but not in the control group.

Using a different methodology the effect of natural progesterone was recently examined

by Gerhard and colleagues.[50] In a small placebo-controlled crossover trial study of postmenopausal women with mild hypercholesterolemia, subjects were randomized to receive transdermal oestradiol, with or without vaginal micronized progesterone. To assess endothelium-dependent vasodilation, brachial artery diameter was determined at baseline and after a flow stimulus induced by reactive hyperemia. During oestradiol therapy, reactive hyperemia caused an 11.1% change in brachial artery diameter compared with 4.7% during placebo therapy ($P < 0.001$). Progesterone did not significantly attenuate this improvement. During combined oestrogen and progesterone therapy, flow-mediated vasodilation of the brachial artery was 9.6%, which was not significantly different from the changes seen with oestradiol alone.

In contrast, in a recent study designed to compare the effects of the C21 progestogen dydrogesterone and the C19 testosterone derivative norethisterone on carotid artery PI Luckas and colleagues[51] found an effect of progestogens on PI. They used a randomized double-blind crossover design and reported that addition of progestogen resulted in a significant increase in the carotid artery PI from a median value of 1.67 during the oestrogen-only phase to 1.77 ($P = 0.02$) during the combined phase. This was seen with both dydrogesterone and norethisterone and there was no significant difference in the size of the effect caused by either progestogen.

The time course of the effects of norethisterone acetate on uterine artery PI has been reported.[52] Nine postmenopausal women were treated with either transdermal 17β-oestradiol 0.1 mg/day or CEE 1.25 mg/day, to which norethisterone acetate 0.7 mg/day was added for 12 days in a single 28 day cycle

of therapy (*see Fig. 7.3.*). Uterine artery PI was measured every 3–5 days over one treatment cycle. Compared with the oestrogen-only phase of the treatment cycle, norethisterone acetate increased the mean uterine artery PI by 30%. Importantly, the PI fell significantly within 4 days of ceasing progestogen.

In summary, several studies support the

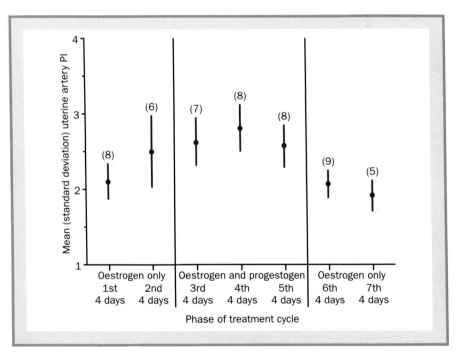

Figure 7.3
Mean (standard deviation) of uterine artery PI of sequential recordings taken during a 28 day cycle of treatment. There was a significant difference in PI between the 1st and 5th phases (P < 0.01); 4th and 6th (P < 0.01); 4th and 7th (P < 0.001); 5th and 6th (P < 0.05); and 5th and 7th (P < 0.001).
All values are antilogs of log-transformed data. (Number of subjects in parentheses.) From reference 52, with permission.

hypothesis that progestogens partially reverse the actions of oestrogens on vascular resistivity, and there is evidence that this effect is shortlived.[52] Regimens of continuous combined HRT, in which oestrogen and progestogen are each given daily, may reduce the beneficial vascular effects of oestrogen on each day of treatment. Such an effect is compatible with the results of the Heart and Estrogen/Progestin Replacement Study (HERS) that used continuous combined HRT. Despite beneficial effects on lipids and lipoproteins there was no reduction in coronary artery disease.

Tibolone

There are little published data on the effects of tibolone on blood flow, and further work is needed. It has been demonstrated that tibolone increases cardiac output without increasing the heart rate, leading to an increase in blood flow through capillaries as well as the larger arteries of the upper extremities.[53,54] In a pilot study, tibolone was reported to reduce exercise-induced myocardial ischemia in postmenopausal women with angina pectoris, comparable to the changes seen with oestrogens.[55] From studies in the cholesterol fat rabbit model for atherosclerosis prevention it appears that tibolone could also preserve the ability of the vessel wall to relax or dilate.[56]

Summary

The evidence for a beneficial effect on CHD risk when oestrogens are used alone as HRT is considerable, but the effects of oestrogens and progestogens are less clear. The recent HERS study puts into doubt the use of continuous combined HRT for the secondary prevention of CHD. It appears that oestrogens reduce vascular resistance to flow, which is likely to be a mechanism for reducing atheroma formation and acute vasospasm. The effect of added progestogen on this mechanism is still uncertain. The androgenicity of a progestogen to a certain extent predicts its effects on serum lipids and lipoproteins. It is not known whether the androgenicity of a progestogen predicts the magnitude of its effects on vascular tone in a similar manner.

References

1. Pilote L, Hlatky MA. Attitudes of women toward hormone therapy and prevention of heart disease. *Am Heart J* 1995; **129**: 1237–1238.

2. Stampfer MJ, Colditz GA. Estrogen replacement therapy and coronary heart disease: a quantitative assessment of the epidemiological evidence. *Preventative Med* 1991; **20**: 47–63.

3. Bush TL, Barrett-Connor E, Cowan LD *et al.* Cardiovascular mortality and noncontraceptive use of estrogen in women: results from the Lipid Research Clinics Program Follow-up Study. *Circulation* 1987; **75**: 1102–1109.

4. Henderson B, Paganini-Hill A, Ross R. Oestrogen replacement therapy and protection from acute myocardial infarction. *Am J Obstet Gynecol* 1988; **159**: 27–31.

5. Persson I, Adami H-O, Bergkvist L *et al.* Risk of endometrial cancer after treatment with oestrogens alone or in conjunction with progestogens: results of a prospective study. *BMJ* 1989; **298**: 147–151.

6. Rosenberg L, Armstrong B, Jick H. Myocardial infarction and oestrogen therapy in postmenopausal women. *New Engl J Med* 1976; **294**: 1256–1259.

7. Rosenberg L, Stone D, Shapiro S *et al.* Noncontraceptive oestrogens and myocardial infarction in young women. *JAMA* 1980; **244**: 339–342.

8. Jick H, Dinan B, Rothman KJ. Noncontraceptive oestrogens and non-fatal myocardial infarction. *JAMA* 1978; **239**: 1407–1408.

9. Pfeffer RI, Whipple GH, Kurosaki TT *et al.* Coronary risk and oestrogen use in postmenopausal women. *Am J Epidemiol* 1978; **107**: 479–487.

10. Bain C, Willett WC, Hennekens CH *et al.* Use of postmenopausal hormones and risk of myocardial infarction. *Circulation* 1981; **64**: 42–46.

11. Ross RK, Paganini-Hill A, Mack TM *et al.* Menopausal oestrogen therapy and protection from ischaemic heart disease. *Lancet* 1981; **i**: 858–860.

12. Stampfer M, Willett W, Colditz G *et al.* A prospective study of postmenopausal estrogen therapy and coronary heart disease. *New Engl J Med* 1985; **313**: 1044–1049.

13. Stampfer MJ, Colditz GA, Willett WC *et al.* Postmenopausal oestrogen therapy and coronary heart disease. Ten year follow up from the Nurses Health Study. *New Engl J Med* 1991; **325**: 756–762.

14. Grodstein F, Stampfer MJ, Manson JE *et al.* Postmenopausal estrogen and progestin use and the risk of cardiovascular disease. *New Engl J Med* 1996; **335**: 453–461.

15. Sullivan JM, Zwagg RV, Lemp GF *et al.* Postmenopausal oestrogen use and coronary atherosclerosis. *Annals of Internal Medicine* 1988; **108**: 358–363.

16. McFarland KF, Boniface ME, Hornung CA *et al.* Risk factors and non contraceptive oestrogen use in women with and without coronary disease. *Am Heart J* 1989; **117**: 1209–1214.

17. Gruchow H, Anderson A, Barboriak J *et al.* Postmenopausal oestrogen and occlusion of coronary arteries. *Am Heart J* 1988; **115**: 954–963.

18. Sullivan JM, Zwagg RV, Lemp GF *et al.* Estrogen replacement and coronary artery disease: effect on survival in postmenopausal women. *Archives Int Med* 1990; **150**: 2557–2562.

19. Hunt K, Vessey M, McPherson K. Mortality in a cohort of long-term users of hormone replacement therapy: an updated analysis. *Br J Obstet Gynaecol* 1990; **97**: 1080–1086.

20. Falkeborn M, Persson I, Adami H-O *et al.* The risk of acute myocardial infarction after oestrogen and oestrogen–progestogen replacement. *Br J Obstet Gynaecol* 1992; **99**: 821–828.

21. Hulley S, Grady D, Bush T *et al.* Heart and Estrogen/Progestin Replacement Study (HERS) research group. Randomized trial of estrogen plus progestin for secondary prevention of coronary heart disease in

postmenopausal women. *JAMA* 1998; **280**: 605–613.

22. Joakimsen O, Bonaa KH, Stensland-Bugge E *et al.* Population-based study of age at menopause and ultrasound assessed carotid atherosclerosis: the Tromso Study. *J Clin Epidemiol* 2000; **53**: 525–530.

23. Wren BG, Routledge DA. The effect of type and dosage of oestrogen on the blood pressure of postmenopausal women. *Maturitas* 1983; **5**: 134–142.

24. Lip GYH, Beevers M, Churchill D *et al.* Hormone replcement therapy and blood pressure in hypertensive women. *J Human Hypertension* 1994; **8**: 491–494.

25. Wren BG, Brown LB, Routledge DA. Differential clinical response to oestrogens after the menopause. *Med J Australia* 1982; **2**: 329.

26. Writing group for the PEPI trial. Effects of estrogen or estrogen/progestin regimens on heart disease risk factors in postmenopausal women: the Postmenopausal Estrogen/Progestin Interventions (PEPI) trial. *JAMA* 1995; **273**: 199–208.

27. Padwick M, Whitehead M, Coffer A *et al.* Demonstration of oestrogen receptor related protein in female tissues. In: Studd JWW, Whitehead MI, eds. *The Menopause.* Oxford: Blackwell Scientific, 1988, 227–233.

28. Steinleitner A, Stanczyk F, Levin J *et al.* Decreased in-vitro production of six-keto-prostaglandin F1 alpha on uterine arteries of postmenopausal women. *Am J Obstet Gynecol* 1989; **161**: 1677–1681.

29. Gisclard V, Millar V, van Houte P. Effects of 17 beta oestradiol on endothelium-dependent responses in the rabbit. *Pharmacol Experimental Therapeutics* 1988; **244**: 19–22.

30. Magness RR, Rosenfeld CR. Local and systemic estradiol-17 beta: effects on uterine and systemic vasodilation. *Am J Physiol* 1989; **256**: E536 E542

31. Rosano GMC, Sarrel PM, Poole-Wilson PA *et al.* Beneficial effects of oestrogen on exercise-induced myocardial ishcaemia in women with coronary artery disease. *Lancet* 1993; **342**: 133–136.

32. Bourne T, Hillard T, Whitehead M *et al.* Evidence for a rapid effect of oestrogens on the arterial status of postmenopausal women. *Lancet* 1990; **335**: 1470–1471.

33. Hillard TC, Bourne TH, Whitehead MI *et al.* Differential effects of transdermal estradiol and sequential progestogens on impedance to flow within the uterine arteries of postmenopausal women. *Fertility & Sterility* 1992; **58**: 959–963.

34. Gangar KF, Vyas S, Whitehead MI *et al.* Pulsatility index in the internal carotid artery is influenced by transdermal estradiol and time since menopause. *Lancet* 1991; **338**: 839–842.

35. Marsh MS, Ross D, Whitcroft SIJ *et al.* Oral oestradiol HRT reduces internal carotid artery pulsatility index in postmenopausal women. *Abstracts Br Menopause Soc* 1994, York.

36. Al-Khalili F, Eriksson M, Landgren BM *et al.* Effect of conjugated estrogen on peripheral flow-mediated vasodilation in postmenopausal women. *Am J Cardiol* 1998; **82**: 215–218.

37. Marsh MS, Ross D, Stevenson JC. Changes in serum lipids, lipoprotein and carotid artery resistance to flow produced by oral or transdermal ERT – a randomized double-blind placebo-controlled study. (In preparation.)

38. Williams J, Adams M, Klopfenstein H. Estrogen modulates responses of

atherosclerotic coronary arteries. *Circulation Res* 1990; **81**: 1680–1687.

39. Collins P, Rosano GMC, Sarrel PM *et al.* 17β-oestradiol attenuates acetyl-choline induced coronary arterial constriction in women but not men with coronary artery disease. *Circulation* 1995; **92**; 24–30.

40. Jiang C, Sarrel P, Poole-Wilson P *et al.* Acute effect of 17β-oestradiol on rabbit artery contractile responses to endothelin-1. *Am J Physiol* 1992; **263**: H271–H275.

41. Jiang C, Poole-Wilson P, Sarrel P *et al.* Effect of 17β-oestradiol on contraction, Ca^{2+} current and intracellular free Ca^{2+} in guinea-pig isolated cardiac myocytes. *Br J Pharmacol* 1992; **106**: 739–749.

42. Jiang C, Sarrel P, Lindsay D *et al.* Endothelium-independent relaxation of rabbit coronary artery by 17β-oestradiol in vitro. *Br J Pharmacol* 1991; **104**: 1033–1037.

42. Lieberman EH, Gerhard MD, Uehata A *et al.* Estrogen improves endothelium-dependent flow-mediated vasodilation in postmenopausal women. *Ann Int Med* 1994; **121**: 936–941.

43. Cambien F, Cousterousse O, Tiret L *et al.* Plasma level and gene polymorphism of angiotensin-converting enzyme in relation to myocardial infarction. *Circulation* 1994; **90**: 669–676.

44. Proudler AJ, Hasib Ahmed AI, Crook D *et al.* Hormone replacement therapy and serum angiotensin-converting-enzyme activity in postmenopausal women. *Lancet* 1995; **89**: 89–90.

45. Hillard TC, Bourne TH, Whitehead MI *et al.* Differential effects of transdermal estradiol and sequential progestogens on impedance to flow within the uterine arteries of postmenopausal women. *Fertility & Sterility* 1992; **58**: 959–963.

46. Darj E, Bakos O, Naessen T *et al.* Ultrasonographic blood flow measurement in the carotid arteries in postmenopausal women. *Gynecolog Obstet Investigation* 1999; **47**(1): 20–25.

47. Penotti M, Farina M, Castiglioni E *et al.* Alteration in the pulsatility index values of the internal carotid and middle cerebral arteries after suspension of postmenopausal hormone replacement therapy: a randomized crossover. *Am J Obstet Gynecol* 1996; **175**: 606–611.

48. Cacciatore B, Paakkari I, Toivonen J *et al.* Randomized comparison of oral and transdermal hormone replacement on carotid and uterine artery resistance to blood flow. *Obstet Gynecol* 1998; **92**: 563–568.

49. Lau TK, Wan D, Yim SF *et al.* Prospective, randomized, controlled study of the effect of hormone replacement therapy on peripheral blood flow velocity in postmenopausal women. *Fertility & Sterility* 1998; **70**: 284–288.

50. Gerhard M, Walsh BW, Tawakol A *et al.* Estradiol therapy combined with progesterone andendothelium-dependent vasodilation in postmenopausal women. *Circulation* 1998; **98**: 1158–1163.

51. Luckas MJ, Gleeve T, Biljan MM *et al.* The effect of progestogens on the carotid artery pulsatility index in postmenopausal women on oestrogen replacement therapy. *Eur J Obstet Gynecol Reprod Biol* 1998; **76**: 221–224.

52. Marsh MS, Bourne TH, Whitehead MI *et al.* The temporal effect of progestogen on the uterine artery pulsatility index in postmenopausal women receiving sequential hormone replacement therapy. *Fertlity & Sterility* 1994; **62**, 771–774.

53. Prelevic GM, Beljic T, Ginsburg J. The effect of tibolone on cardiac flow in postmenopausal

women with non insulin dependent diabetes mellitus. *Maturitas* 1997; **27**: 85–90.

54. Hänggi W *et al.* Microscopic findings of the nailfold capillaries—dependence on menopausal status and hormone replacement therapy. *Maturitas* 1995; **22**: 37–46.

55. Lloyd GW, Patel NR, McGing EA *et al.* Acute effects of hormone replacement with

tibolone on myocardial ischemia in women with angina. *Int J Clin Pract* 1998; **52**: 155–157.

56. Zandberg P, Peters JL, Demacker PN *et al.* Tibolone prevents atherosclerotic lesion formation in cholesterol-fed ovariectomized rabbits. *Arterioscler Thromb Vasc Biol* 1998; **18**: 1844–1854.

Hormone replacement therapy and carbohydrate metabolism

John C Stevenson

8

Cardiovascular disease incidence increases with age in women as well as in men, but in women there is an additional increase owing to the menopause.[1] Indeed, women have more than a three-fold increase in risk of atherosclerosis after a natural menopause.[2] Cardiovascular disease is the leading cause of death in women, and loss of ovarian hormones at the menopause is a major risk factor for this disease, particularly coronary heart disease (CHD).[1,3,4] Loss of ovarian function results in an increase in various CHD risk factors which form a metabolic syndrome.[5] These include adverse changes in lipids and lipoproteins, glucose and insulin metabolism, body fat distribution, coagulation and fibrinolysis, an increase in uric acid, and deterioration in vascular endothelial function. There appears to be a clustering of metabolic risk factors in patients with CHD, and it has been proposed that insulin resistance and hyperinsulinaemia are pivotal disturbances.[6,7] Hormone replacement therapy (HRT) might therefore be expected to reverse these changes, thereby reducing the increased cardiovascular disease risk.

Insulin resistance and CHD risk

Insulin resistance is tissue resistance to insulin action, whether this is in terms of glucose or lipid metabolism, or the vasodilatory actions of insulin. Insulin resistance is usually accompanied by hyperinsulinaemia. Insulin promotes smooth muscle cell proliferation and arterial lipid deposition, and hence may be involved in the pathogenesis of atheroma.[8]

Insulin resistance has conventionally been defined as the change in glucose elimination rate elicited by a unit change in insulin concentration. It is difficult to quantitate, and only two methods used in clinical practice provide a true measure of insulin sensitivity (the inverse of insulin resistance).[9] These are the euglycaemic hyperinsulinaemic clamp and the minimal model analysis of glucose and insulin profiles obtained during an intravenous glucose tolerance test (IVGTT), and the two methods correlate closely with each other.[10] The euglycaemic hyperinsulinaemic clamp utilizes a constant intravenous infusion of insulin and a varying intravenous infusion of glucose. Though it gives a true estimate of insulin sensitivity, the method is extremely labour intensive and time consuming, and it is also non-physiological. The minimal model utilizes the non-steady-state glucose and insulin responses to an intravenous glucose bolus to provide a measure of the constant that best relates change in glucose elimination to change in insulin concentration in the plasma. Although the clinical technique is straightforward, and the insulin response is physiological, the mathematical modelling is complex and requires skilled and experienced operators. Furthermore, this technique may not be valid in diabetics. A number of surrogates for the assessment of insulin resistance have been proposed and used, but they do not accurately reflect true insulin sensitivity, which greatly limits their usefulness. For example, decreases in fasting glucose and insulin concentrations are often interpreted as reflecting reduced insulin resistance, yet they may actually reflect the opposite.[11]

The effects of sex hormone deficiency and replacement on glucose and insulin metabolism may be of considerable importance for CHD risk. Diabetic women have a higher incidence of CHD than diabetic men,[12] and mortality from ischaemic heart disease in diabetic women is increased three-fold compared with non-diabetics.[13] Apart from frank diabetes, lesser degrees of glucose intolerance are still predictive of subsequent CHD (Welborn and Wearne, 1979; Jarrett et al, 1982; Fuller et al, 1983; Donahue et al, 1987).[14–17] Protein glycosylation is a possible mechanism linking elevated glucose levels with CHD in diabetics, but the increased risk seen in those with lesser degrees of glucose tolerance is more likely to be mediated through insulin resistance and hyperinsulinaemia. Elevated insulin concentrations are frequently found in both men and women with coronary heart disease,[18,19] and appear to be owed to insulin resistance.[19] We have also demonstrated increased insulin resistance in both men[20] and women[21] with cardiological syndrome X.

Hyperinsulinaemia may increase CHD risk by directly promoting atherogenesis, and insulin propeptides may be of importance in this respect.[22] However, increased insulin concentrations may adversely affect several other CHD risk factors. There is an association between hyperinsulinaemia and hypertension,[23] and we have found a positive relationship between insulin resistance and blood pressure.[24] Insulin stimulates renal sodium reabsorption and has a sympathomimetic effect, which will tend to raise blood pressure. Normally, these effects might be counteracted by insulin-induced vasodilatation, but in insulin-resistant states this compensatory mechanism is impaired.[25] Indeed, we have demonstrated that an intravenous glucose bolus, which stimulates endogenous insulin secretion, results in increased forearm blood flow in normals, yet there is a paradoxical decrease in patients with CHD, who tend to be insulin resistant.[26]

Insulin resistance and hyperinsulinaemia are also related to adverse changes in lipids and lipoproteins such as increased triglycerides and reduced high density lipoproteins (HDL) or HDL_2 concentrations.[19] Furthermore,

hyperinsulinaemia is associated with increased proportions of small dense low density lipoproteins (LDL).[27] These particles are less readily cleared by the $apoB_{100}$ receptors, and are more open to oxidative damage. Additionally, glycated LDL are also more likely to be cleared from the circulation by scavenger mechanisms rather than by the $apoB_{100}$ receptors. Thus patients with impaired glucose tolerance are likely to produce more atherogenic lipoproteins. These changes in lipids and lipoproteins will augment the adverse changes seen as a result of the menopause itself. These include increases in total cholesterol, triglycerides, and LDL, and decreases in HDL and HDL_2.[28] There are also increases in lipoprotein (a) and perhaps decreases in the clearance of atherogenic particles.

This association of adverse CHD risk factors, with insulin resistance a pivotal mechanism, is now termed the 'insulin resistance' syndrome or 'metabolic' syndrome, and there are various other components (*Table 8.1*). These include increased levels of the anti-fibrinolytic plasminogen activator inhibitor-1 (PAI-1),[29] increased proportions of android (central or upper body segment) fat,[30] and increased leptin concentrations.[31]

Table 8.1
Some proposed manifestations and associations of the insulin resistance syndrome.

Insulin resistance
Hyperinsulinaemia
Increased proportion of insulin
    propeptides
Impaired glucose tolerance
Increased triglycerides
Decreased HDL and HDL_2 cholesterol
Increased proportion of small dense
    LDL cholesterol
Increased proportion of android fat
Increased NEFA* flux
Increased plasminogen activator
    inhibitor-1
Decreased tissue plasminogen activator
Increased leptin
Decreased arterial wall compliance
Increased blood pressure
Decreased arterial blood flow

Non-esterified fatty acids.

Effect of menopause on glucose and insulin metabolism

Few studies have investigated changes in glucose and insulin metabolism in relation to the menopause. One longitudinal study of women going through natural menopause showed increases in fasting glucose and insulin concentrations, but these were also seen in those women who remained premenopausal, suggesting an effect of ageing.[32] We studied glucose and insulin metabolism in 86 healthy postmenopausal women who underwent an intravenous glucose tolerance test with measurement of glucose, insulin, and C-peptide concentrations.[33] No relationship was seen between either chronological age or menopausal age and any glucose or C-peptide parameters, although body mass index was related to fasting glucose and post-glucose challenge glucose area. We found a positive and independent relationship between menopausal age and both fasting insulin concentration and post-glucose challenge insulin area, but no relationship between these parameters and chronological age. This clearly shows that following the menopause there is a progressive rise in insulin concentrations and responses to glucose challenge. In another study of 158 premenopausal and postmenopausal women, we performed mathematical modelling analyses of the plasma concentration profiles of glucose, insulin, and C-peptide in response to an intravenous glucose challenge to obtain measures of insulin sensitivity, secretion, and elimination.[34] We found that postmenopausal women had a reduction in pancreatic insulin secretion which was counterbalanced by a reduction in insulin elimination (*Fig. 8.1*). Although insulin sensitivity did not differ between premenopausal and postmenopausal women, it decreased progressively with age in the postmenopausal women (*Fig. 8.2*), indicating a progressive increase in insulin

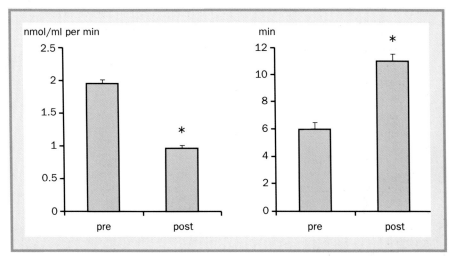

Figure 8.1
*Effect of menopause on pancreatic insulin secretion and insulin elimination (+SEM). *P < 0.001. From reference 34, with permission.*

resistance. A recent smaller study of 83 premenopausal and postmenopausal women similarly showed no difference between the two groups of women in terms of insulin sensitivity as assessed by the euglycaemic hyperinsulinaemic clamp technique.[35] One possible reason for the apparent lack of a menopause effect on insulin sensitivity in these two studies is that both studied premenopausal women in the luteal phase of the menstrual cycle, when oestradiol levels are lower, and it is possible that insulin sensitivity is lower in this phase of the cycle. This would tend to mask any differences in insulin

sensitivity in comparisons between premenopausal and postmenopausal women.

In another much smaller study, there was some evidence that postmenopausal women had lower insulin sensitivity values than premenopausal women as assessed by the IVGTT with modelling analyses.[36]

In summary, it would appear that the menopause is associated with reduced pancreatic insulin secretion but also with reduced insulin elimination, thereby resulting in little change in circulating insulin concentrations. The progressive rise in insulin concentrations observed thereafter appears to

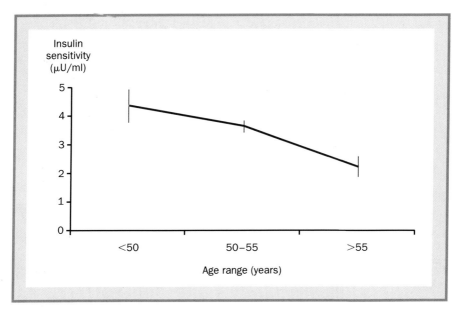

Figure 8.2
Effect of age on insulin sensitivity (+SEM) in postmenopausal women. From reference 34, with permission.

result from the progressive increase in insulin resistance seen after the menopause. Postmenopausal women thus become increasingly insulin resistant and hyperinsulinaemic.

HRT effects on glucose and insulin metabolism

Experimental studies both *in vitro* and *in vivo* have demonstrated increased pancreatic

insulin secretion in response to oestrogen or progesterone administration. However, whereas oestradiol decreases insulin resistance, progesterone appears to increase it.

Clinical studies of the effects of 17β-oestradiol in postmenopausal women suggest an improvement in insulin resistance.[37,38] Progestogen addition, which is necessary in HRT given to non-hysterectomized women, may produce certain adverse effects on glucose and insulin metabolism. Alkylated oestrogens such as ethinyl oestradiol and conjugated equine oestrogens may raise insulin levels and impair glucose tolerance.[39]

The postmenopausal oestrogen/progestogen intervention (PEPI) study showed a decrease in fasting glucose and insulin levels with conjugated equine oestrogens, with or without progestogen addition.[40] However, following an oral glucose challenge, glucose concentrations were increased by the HRT. As stated above, it is difficult to draw any meaningful conclusions from such surrogate markers of insulin resistance. A small study using another surrogate for insulin resistance, the insulin tolerance test, has previously shown a possible bimodal effect of conjugated equine oestrogens on insulin sensitivity, with a lower dose of 0.625 mg/day improving it whereas a higher dose of 1.25 mg/day caused a deterioration (Lindheim *et al*, 1993). The addition of medroxyprogesterone acetate also caused a deterioration.

We performed a study in healthy postmenopausal women comparing two different HRT regimens against no treatment.[42] One regimen used oral conjugated equine oestrogens 0.625 mg daily with the cyclical addition of *dl*-norgestrel 0.15 mg daily, whereas the other comprised transdermal 17β-oestradiol 0.05 mg daily together with cyclical norethisterone acetate 0.25 mg daily. Transdermal treatment had no significant effect on glucose tolerance or insulin concentrations. In contrast, oral therapy caused a reduction in the initial plasma insulin response to intravenous glucose, which in turn resulted in a reduction in glucose elimination rate at the outset of the test and an overall elevation in glucose concentrations. These changes increased the stimulation of pancreatic insulin secretion and hence the overall insulin response during the test. Both treatments were associated with increased hepatic insulin uptake, but an increase in first phase pancreatic insulin secretion compensated for this in the transdermal group. In the oral group, a significant increase in insulin resistance was seen during the combined oestrogen/progestin phase of treatment compared with the oestrogen-alone phase, whereas no changes were seen with transdermal therapy.

The fact that transdermal 17β-oestradiol was not associated with a reduction in insulin resistance, which might have been expected, could have owed to such an effect being negated by the norethisterone acetate, with this negative effect of norethisterone acetate carried over into the oestrogen-alone phase of treatment. This concept is supported by our findings from a further study in which we compared the effects of 17β-oestradiol given either orally or transdermally, together with cyclical oral norethisterone acetate over 12 months.[43] Insulin sensitivity, secretion, and elimination were assessed using modelling of IVGTT parameters. Insulin sensitivity was

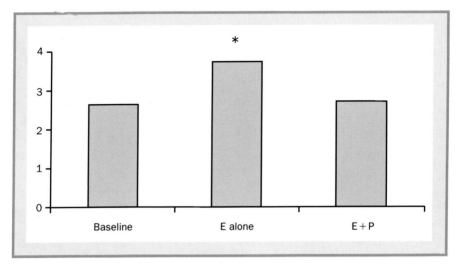

Figure 8.3
*Insulin sensitivity in postmenopausal women receiving oral 17β-oestradiol 2 mg daily with cyclical oral norethisterone acetate 1 mg daily. Changes are shown at baseline, during the oestrogen-alone phase (E), and in the combined oestrogen/progestogen phase (E + P). *P < 0.05. From reference 43, with permission.*

increased by the oral 17β-oestradiol, but this was reversed by the addition of norethisterone acetate (*Fig. 8.3*). Transdermal 17β-oestradiol again had no effect on insulin sensitivity. Both treatments were associated with an increase in insulin secretion and hepatic insulin uptake. A small 6-month study of transdermal oestradiol without the systemic addition of a progestogen was able to demonstrate an improvement in insulin sensitivity as assessed by an insulin tolerance test. In contrast, a study using the clamp technique did not demonstrate any change in insulin sensitivity in women receiving transdermal oestradiol alone, or after the addition of oral norethisterone.[44] However, the study duration was extremely short, only 6 weeks. A study of high or low dose continuous combined oral oestradiol and norethisterone acetate using the clamp technique demonstrated a deterioration in insulin sensitivity with the high dose (oestradiol 2 mg, norethisterone acetate 1 mg) which was not seen with the low dose (oestradiol 1 mg, norethisterone 0.5 mg).[45]

The use of a non-androgenic progestogen

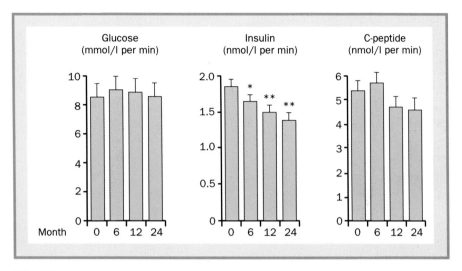

Figure 8.4
*Incremental glucose, insulin, and C-peptide responses (+SEM) to an oral glucose challenge during combined phase of treatment in postmenopausal women receiving oral 17β-oestradiol 2 mg daily with cyclical dydrogesterone 10 mg daily. *P < 0.05, **P < 0.01. From reference 46, with permission.*

may avoid these adverse changes in glucose and insulin metabolism. We studied the effects of oral administration of 17β-oestradiol and cyclical dydrogesterone on glucose and insulin metabolism using oral glucose tolerance testing.[46] Mean fasting glucose and C-peptide concentrations and post-glucose challenge incremental glucose and C-peptide areas remained unchanged during the study whereas the fasting insulin concentration and post-glucose challenge response fell significantly (*Fig. 8.4*). These findings are consistent with an improvement in insulin resistance and insulin elimination with this regimen. In a recent study using the clamp technique, transdermal oestradiol with the addition of cyclical dydrogesterone resulted in an increase in insulin sensitivity and in hepatic insulin uptake.[47]

The effect of HRT in women with diabetes mellitus seems also to be beneficial. Women with non-insulin-dependent diabetes mellitus taking oral 17β-oestradiol with cyclical norethisterone acetate in a randomized placebo-controlled crossover study showed improvements in glucose homeostasis, including glycosylated haemoglobin.[48] Similar findings were seen in a similar study of shorter duration.[49] Tibolone, a synthetic steroid with oestrogenic, progestogenic, and androgenic properties, has also been shown to have no adverse effects in a short-term study of postmenopausal non-insulin-dependent diabetic women.[50] Both oral 17β-oestradiol and tibolone have also produced some beneficial effects in lipids and lipoproteins in diabetic women,[49,50] suggesting further benefit in terms of CHD risk.

Conclusions

There is little doubt that the metabolic disturbances seen following the loss of ovarian function are most important in the development of cardiovascular disease in women. The loss of hormones at the menopause appears to reduce both insulin secretion and elimination, but increasing insulin resistance thereafter brings about an increase in circulating insulin concentrations. Changes in lipids and lipoproteins are in an adverse direction, as are changes in body fat distribution and haemostatic factors. These adverse changes are likely to be particularly harmful to women with diabetes mellitus who are already at increased risk for CHD.

Hormone replacement therapy with oestrogen alone appears to improve most of the metabolic abnormalities related to the menopause, but this depends in part on the type of oestrogen used and the route of administration. 17β-Oestradiol, both oral and to a lesser extent transdermal, improves insulin sensitivity, secretion, and elimination. Conjugated equine oestrogens, particularly at higher doses, have less favourable effects. The addition of progestogen may influence the metabolic changes induced by oestrogens, and this varies according to the type of the progestogen. The more androgenic progestogens, such as norgestrel and norethisterone, tend to reverse the beneficial effects of oestrogens, as does the less androgenic medroxyprogesterone acetate. In contrast, dydrogesterone appears to have little negative impact on oestrogenic effects. Overall, the metabolic effects of any of the current HRT regimens, including tibolone, seem likely to be beneficial for CHD in non-diabetic women. However, HRT regimens should be tailored to produce the most favourable changes in metabolic risk factors in postmenopausal women at increased risk for CHD, particularly those with diabetes mellitus, for whom the potential for benefit is considerable.

References

1. Gordon T, Kannel WB, Hjortland MC *et al*. Menopause and coronary heart disease. The Framingham Study. *Ann Int Med* 1978; **89**: 157–161.

2. Witteman JCM, Grobbee DE, Kok FJ *et al*.

Increased risk of atherosclerosis in women after the menopause. *Br Med J* 1989; **298**: 642–644.

3. Oliver MF, Boyd GS. Effect of bilateral ovariectomy on coronary artery disease and serum lipid levels. *Lancet* 1959; **ii**: 690–692.

4. Sznajderman M, Oliver MF. Spontaneous premature menopause, ischaemic heart disease and serum lipids. *Lancet* 1963; **i**: 962–964.

5. Spencer CP, Godsland IF, Stevenson JC. Is there a menopausal metabolic syndrome? *Gynaecol Endocrinol* 1997; **11**: 341–355.

6. Reaven GM. Role of insulin resistance in human disease. *Diabetes* 1988; **37**: 1595–1607.

7. Godsland IF, Stevenson JC. Insulin resistance: syndrome or tendency? *Lancet* 1995; **346**: 100–103.

8. Stout R. Insulin and atheroma: 20-yr perspective. *Diabetes Care* 1990; **13**: 631–654.

9. Stevenson JC, Godsland IF. Insulin resistance and coronary heart disease. *Risk* 1997; **5**: 4–8.

10. Swan JW, Walton C, Godsland IF. Assessment of insulin sensitivity in man: a comparison of minimal model and euglycaemic clamp derived measures in health and heart failure. *Clin Sci* 1994; **86**: 317–322.

11. Bruce R, Lees B, Whitcroft SIJ *et al.* Changes in body composition with danazol therapy. *Fertil Steril* 1991; **56**: 574–576.

12. Abbott W, Lillioja S, Young A. Relationships between plasma lipoprotein concentrations and insulin action in an obese hyperinsulinaemic population. *Diabetes* 1987; **36**: 897–904.

13. Barrett-Connor EL, Cohn BA, Wingard DL *et al.* Why is diabetes mellitus a stronger risk factor for fatal ischaemic heart disease in women than men? *J Am Med Assoc* 1991; **265**: 627–631.

14. Welborn TA, Wearne K. Coronary heart disease incidence and cardiovascular mortality in Busselton with reference to glucose and insulin concentrations. *Diabetes Care* 1979; **2**: 154–160.

15. Jarrett RJ, McCartney P, Keen H. The Bedford Survey: ten year mortality rates in newly diagnosed diabetics, borderline diabetics and normoglycaemic controls and risk for coronary heart disease in borderline diabetics. *Diabetologia* 1982; **22**: 79–84.

16. Fuller JH, Shipley MJ, Rose G *et al.* Mortality from coronary heart disease and stroke in relation to degree of glycaemia: the Whitehall Study. *Br Med J* 1983; **287**: 867–870.

17. Donahue RP, Abbott RD, Reed DM *et al.* Post-challenge glucose concentration and coronary heart disease in men of Japanese ancestry. *Diabetes* 1987; **36**: 689–692.

18. Rönnemaa T, Laakso M, Pyörälä K *et al.* High fasting plasma insulin is an indicator of coronary heart disease in non-insulin-dependent diabetic patients and non-diabetic subjects. *Arteriosclerosis* 1991; **11**: 80–90.

19. Ley CJ, Swan J, Godsland IF *et al.* Insulin resistance, lipoproteins, body fat and hemostasis in non-obese males with angina and normal or abnormal coronary angiograms. *J Am Coll Cardiol* 1994; **23**: 377–383.

20. Swan JW, Walton C, Godsland IF *et al.* The insulin resistance syndrome as a feature of cardiological syndrome X in non-obese men. *Br Heart J* 1994; **71**: 41–44.

21. Godsland IF, Crook D, Stevenson JC *et al.* Insulin resistance syndrome in postmenopausal women with cardiological syndrome X. *Br Heart J* 1995; **74**: 47–52.

22. Båvenholm P, Proudler AJ, Tornvall P et al. Insulin, intact and split proinsulin and coronary artery disease in young men. Circulation 1995; 92: 1422–1429.

23. Ferrannini E, Buzziogli G, Bonadonna R et al. Insulin resistance in essential hypertension. N Engl J Med 1987; 317: 350–357.

24. Walton C, Lees B, Godsland IF et al. Relationship between insulin metabolism, serum lipid profile, body fat distribution and blood pressure in healthy men. Atherosclerosis 1995; 118: 35–43.

25. Baron AD. Hemodynamic actions of insulin. Am J Physiol 1994; 267: E187–E202.

26. Leyva F, Rauchaus M, Anker SD et al. Non-invasive assessment of vascular function. Paradoxical vascular response to intravenous glucose in coronary heart disease. Eur Heart J 2000; 21: 39–44.

27. Krauss RM. The tangled web of coronary risk factors. Am J Med 1991; 90(suppl 2A): 36–41.

28. Stevenson JC, Crook D, Godsland IF. Influence of age and menopause on serum lipids and lipoproteins in healthy women. Atherosclerosis 1993; 98: 83–90.

29. Juhan-Vague I, Alessi MC, Joly P et al. Plasma plasminogen activator inhibitor 1 in angina pectoris. Influence of plasma insulin and acute-phase response. Arteriosclerosis 1989; 9: 362–367.

30. Stevenson JC, Lees B, Bruce R et al. Influence of body composition on lipid metabolism in postmenopausal women. In: Christiansen C, Overgaard K, eds. Osteoporosis 1990. Copenhagen: Osteopress ApS, 1990, 1837–1838.

31. Leyva F, Godsland IF, Ghatei M et al. Hyperleptinaemia as a component of a metabolic syndrome of cardiovascular risk. Arteriosclerosis Thromb Vasc Biol 1998; 18: 928–933.

32. Matthews KA, Meilahn E, Kuller LH et al. Menopause and risk factors for coronary heart disease. N Engl J Med 1989; 321: 641–646.

33. Proudler AJ, Felton CV, Stevenson JC. Ageing and the response of plasma insulin, glucose and C-peptide concentrations to intravenous glucose in postmenopausal women. Clinical Science 1992; 83: 489–494.

34. Walton C, Godsland IF, Proudler AJ et al. The effects of the menopause on insulin sensitivity, secretion and elimination in non-obese, healthy women. Eur J Clin Invest 1993; 23: 466–473.

35. Toth MJ, Sites CK, Eltabbakh GH et al. Effect of menopausal status on insulin-stimulated glucose disposal: comparison of middle-aged premenopausal and early postmenopausal women. Diabetes Care 2000; 23: 801–806.

36. Lindheim SR, Buchanan TA, Duffy DM et al. Comparison of estimates of insulin sensitivity in pre- and postmenopausal women using the insulin tolerance test and the frequently sampled intravenous glucose tolerance test. J Soc Gynecol Investig 1994; 1: 150–154.

37. Notelovitz M, Johnston M, Smith S et al. Metabolic and hormonal effects of 25 mg and 50 mg 17β estradiol implants in surgically menopausal women. Obstet Gynecol 1987; 70: 749–754.

38. Cagnacci A, Soldani R, Carriero PL et al. Effects of low doses of transdermal 17β-estradiol on carbohydrate metabolism in postmenopausal women. J Clin Endocrinol Metab 1992; 74: 1396–1400.

39. Spellacy WN, Buhi WC, Birk SA. The effects of estrogens on carbohydrate metabolism:

glucose, insulin and growth hormone studies on one hundred and seventy one women ingesting Premarin, mestranol and ethinyl estradiol for six months. *Am J Obstet Gynecol* 1972; **114**: 378–392.

40. Espeland MA, Hogan PE, Fineberg SE *et al.* Effect of postmenopausal hormone therapy on glucose and insulin concentrations. PEPI Investigators. Postmenopausal Estrogen/ Progesti Interventions. *Diabetes Care* 1998; **21**: 1589–1595.

41. Lindheim SR, Presser SC, Ditkoff EC *et al.* A possible bimodal effect of estrogen on insulin sensitivity in postmenopausal women and the attenuating effect of added progestin. *Fertil Steril* 1993; **60**: 664–667.

42. Godsland IF, Gangar KF, Walton C *et al.* Insulin resistance, secretion, and elimination in postmenopausal women receiving oral or transdermal hormone replacement therapy. *Metabolism* 1993; **42**: 846–853.

43. Spencer CP, Godsland IF, Cooper AJ *et al.* Effects of oral and transdermal 17β-estradiol with cyclical oral norethindrone acetate on insulin sensitivity, secretion, and elimination in postmenopausal women. *Metabolism* 2000; **49**: 742–747.

44. Duncan AC, Lyall H, Roberts RN *et al.* The effect of estradiol and a combined estradiol/ progestagen preparation on insulin sensitivity in healthy postmenopausal women. *J Clin Endocrinol Metab* 1999; **84**: 2402–2407.

45. Kimmerle R, Heinemann L, Heise T *et al.* Influence of continuous combined estradiol- norethisterone acetate preparations on insulin sensitivity in postmenopausal nondiabetic women. *Menopause* 1999; **6**: 36–42.

46. Crook D, Godsland IF, Hull J *et al.* Hormone replacement therapy with dydrogesterone and oestradiol-17β: effects on serum lipoproteins and glucose tolerance. *Br J Obstet Gynaecol* 1997; **104**: 298–304.

47. Cucinelli F, Paparella P, Soranna L *et al.* Differential effect of transdermal estrogen plus progestagen replacement therapy on insulin metabolism in postmenopausal women: relation to their insulinemic secretion. *Eur J Endocrinol* 1999; **140**: 215–223.

48. Andersson B, Mattsson LA, Hahn L *et al.* Estrogen replacement therapy decreases hyperandrogenicity and improves glucose homeostasis and plasma lipids in postmenopausal women with noninsulin- dependent diabetes mellitus. J Clin Endocrinol Metab 1997; **82**: 638–643.

49. Brussaard HE, Gevers Leuven JA *et al.* Short term oestrogen replacement therapy improves insulin resistance, lipids and fibrinolysis in postmenopausal women with NIDDM. *Diabetologia* 1997; **40**: 843–849.

50. Feher MD, Cox A, Levy A *et al.* Short term blood pressure and metabolic effects of tibolone in postmenopausal women with non insulin dependent diabetes. *Br J Obstet Gynaecol* 1996; **103**: 281–283.

Hormone replacement therapy, stroke and thromboembolism: epidemiological evidence

Anette Tønnes Pedersen, Bent Ottesen

9

For the last decades there has been increasing epidemiological evidence that postmenopausal treatment with sex steroids in physiological doses may reduce the relative risk of cardiovascular disease (CVD).[1] When analysing the influence of hormone replacement therapy (HRT) on the risk of cardiovascular events it is important to bear in mind that CVD comprises pathogenically different diseases, arterial as well as venous, and that the aetiology of thromboembolic diseases is multifactorial.

On the arterial side, the most prominent heart diseases are angina pectoris and acute myocardial infarction due to thrombosis, often associated with atherosclerosis. Cerebral infarctions, or stroke, are commonly considered atherothrombotic or cardioembolic. Transient ischaemic attacks are most common in patients with large artery atherothrombotic disease. Less common causes include hypercoagulable states.

On the venous side, the majority of the thromboembolic events take place in the pulmonary veins or in the deep veins in the lower extremities. The venous diseases are often caused by an imbalance in the haemostatic factors towards a hypercoagulative state.

Numerous epidemiological studies support the notion that postmenopausal use of HRT is associated with a 40–60% reduction in the risk of coronary heart disease and a 2–4-fold increased risk of venous thromboembolism, while it has a neutral effect on the risk of stroke. There is therefore no simple answer to the question of a possible protective effect of HRT on the risk of thrombosis. This chapter will deal with the epidemiological evidence.

Observational studies

Analytic epidemiology examines the determinants of a specific disease by testing the hypotheses formulated from associations found in descriptive studies, with the ultimate goal of judging whether a particular exposure causes or prevents disease. The two basic types of observational analytic investigations are the case-control and the cohort design – each offering advantages and disadvantages. The decision to use a particular design strategy is based on features of the exposure and disease, the current state of knowledge and logistic considerations such as available time and resources.

In the case-control study, cases and controls are selected on the basis of presence or absence of the disease of interest (e.g. CVD). The exposure of interest is then compared between the two groups. In contrast, the subjects for a cohort study are classified on the basis of presence or absence of exposure to the factor of interest and compared with respect to the subsequent development of disease. The cohort study is therefore considered to be a 'prospective' design, while the case-control study often is designated as 'retrospective'.

Case-control studies are especially efficient in terms of both time and costs relative to other analytic approaches, as data collection is based on cases which have already been diagnosed with the disease of interest. Case-control studies are well suited to the evaluation of rare diseases or diseases with long latent periods. An important difficulty with case-control studies is that both the exposure and disease have already occurred at the time the participants enter into the study. This design is therefore particularly susceptible to bias from the differential selection of cases and controls and bias due to recall.

The prospective cohort design determines the temporal relationship between exposure and disease and minimizes bias in the ascertainment of exposure. Cohort studies are often extremely time-consuming and the validity of the results can be seriously affected by losses to follow-up.

Intervention studies or clinical trials may be viewed as a type of prospective cohort study as participants are identified on the basis of their exposure status, randomized or non-randomized, and followed to determine whether they develop the disease or not.

A prominent concern in assessments of the influence of HRT in observational studies is that hormone users, as a self-selected group, are different both from former-users and from never-users.[2] Women taking oestrogen seem to have more favourable lifestyles regarding heart disease risk factors – the 'healthy user effect'. Until recently, women with less favourable cardiovascular risk profiles due to hypertension, diabetes or present ischaemic heart disease, were less likely to be prescribed HRT due to contraindications listed on the oestrogen preparation by the manufacturer. It is also possible that potential unknown confounders not included in previous analyses could be associated with the use of HRT and also be strong predictors of CVD. Such an influence cannot be excluded, although it does not seem likely.

When the possible causal relationship of a protective effect of HRT on the risk of CVD is evaluated, consistency with other investigations, strength of the association, time sequence between exposure and event, possible dose–response relationships and biologic credibility should all be taken into consideration.

HRT and stroke

Stroke is the common name for a group of cerebrovascular diseases characterized by sudden onset of neurological deficit, including cerebral infarction, intracerebral haemorrhage and subarachnoid haemorrhage. It is often difficult to establish the pathogenesis of a stroke from clinical observations only. Computed tomography or magnetic resonance imaging enables differentiation between thromboembolic and haemorrhagic disorders. Cerebral infarctions are commonly considered atherothrombotic or cardioembolic. The incidence rate of a first-ever stroke among women aged 45–64 years is 1–2 per 1000 per year.[3]

Whereas the existing data on the protective effect of oestrogen replacement therapy on the risk of coronary heart disease have been compelling, the data on the effect of HRT on the risk of stroke have for a long time remained controversial. A major difficulty when reviewing the literature is the lack of discrimination between haemorrhagic and thromboembolic incidents. Increased as well as decreased risk of stroke in women using oestrogen replacement therapy have been reported. Many of the studies performed have not been able to detect any effect of hormone use on the risk of stroke due to a low number of cases.

Figure 9.1 gives an overview of the results of the better quality studies published.[4, 5–15] Overall, there seems to be a neutral effect of HRT on the risk of ischaemic stroke. All of the cohort studies that have assessed the influence of HRT on stroke *mortality* have,

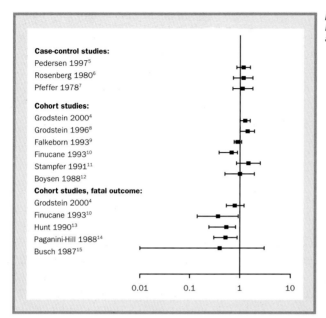

Figure 9.1
Risk of ischaemic stroke
according to use of HRT

however, shown a protective effect of ever-use of HRT, although not all have been statistically significant. This finding could be explained by a reduction in case fatality due to the influence of HRT.

The latest update from the Nurses Health Study with follow-up from 1976 to 1996, based on 432 ischaemic stroke cases, revealed a significantly increased risk of thromboembolic stroke in current users of HRT compared with never-users, RR 1.26 (95% CI, 1.00–1.61). For death due to stroke, the relative risk was 0.81 (95% CI, 0.54–1.22).[4]

The largest study on this subject so far is the Danish case-control study, including a total of 1422 stroke cases – among those were 846 thromboembolic events and 321 cases of transient ischaemic attacks.[5] After adjustment for confounding factors, no significant associations were detected between non-fatal thromboembolic infarction and either current use of unopposed oestrogen replacement therapy, OR 1.16 (95% CI, 0.86–1.58), or current use of combined oestrogen-progestogen therapy, OR 1.17 (95% CI, 0.92–1.47). However, a two-fold significantly increased risk of transient ischaemic attacks was found among women who were at the time using unopposed oestrogens, OR 2.11 (95% CI, 1.41–3.17). This finding could support the hypothesis of a reduction in case fatality due to the influence of HRT, found in other observational studies. HRT users are not necessarily protected from cerebrovascular incidents, but do experience milder forms and are therefore less likely to die from them. One would therefore expect to find an overall unchanged risk of stroke, including transient ischaemic attacks, but an altered distribution with fewer fatal stroke events and more cases of transient ischaemic attacks among HRT users than among non-users. These results therefore do not exclude a possible protection of oestrogen therapy against fatal stroke events.

HRT and venous thromboembolism

In 1996 four studies on HRT and risk of venous thromboembolism (VTE) were published in the same issue of the *Lancet*, all revealing a 2–4-fold increase in the risk of pulmonary embolism or deep vein thromboembolism.[16–19] Two additional surveys have been published subsequently.[20–21] The results are given in *Figure 9.2*.

It is important to note that in four of the six studies, the risk was highest among short-term current users (4–6-fold higher),

especially within the first year of therapy. No increased risk was found among former hormone users. These findings suggest an influence of HRT on a pathway or pathways with fairly rapid effect. No obvious differences were found between users of high or low doses of oestrogen or between users of unopposed oestrogen or combined oestrogen–progestogen replacement therapy.

Hepatic expression of the genes for several coagulation and fibrinolytic proteins is regulated by oestrogen through oestrogen receptors.[22] Continuous oestrogen therapy is associated with decreased plasma fibrinogen concentrations and decreased concentrations of the anticoagulant protein antithrombin III, but also with a decrease in plasma concentrations of the antifibrinolytic protein plasminogen-activator inhibitor type 1. The net effect of oestrogen on coagulation and fibrinolysis depends on the form of oestrogen used, as well as the dose and the duration of therapy. HRT could initially very well lead to a hypercoagulative state accounting for the increased risk of VTE during the first year of therapy in predisposed subjects.

In clinical counselling it is important to emphasize that the incidence of VTE is very low, occurring in only 1–2 per 10,000 women per year.[20] The *absolute* risk of VTE associated with HRT is therefore extremely small, resulting in 1–2 additional cases per 10,000 women per year.

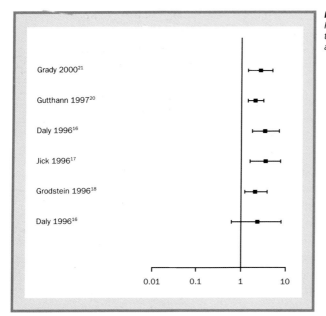

Figure 9.2
Risk of venous thromboembolism according to use of HRT

Conclusions

Oestrogen has multiple potentially beneficial effects on the cardiovascular system, which could explain the overall reduced risk in morbidity and mortality from cardiovascular disease observed in hormone-substituted postmenopausal women. The diverse effects of oestrogen on arterial and venous thromboembolic events could be explained by the endothelium-protective effects and the direct beneficial effects on the vessel wall, on the one hand, and the pro-coagulative effects of oestrogens, on the other hand. More studies are needed to clarify whether the acute vascular changes induced by HRT translate into long-term benefit.

Randomized trials are in general required to determine if findings from observational studies are biased by confounding, selection or compliance. The question whether the hypothesis of a protective effect of HRT on the cardiovascular system, as strongly suggested by the large amount of observational data available, will be elucidated by ongoing randomized clinical trials. However, it should be remembered that the fact that a trial is carried out in one group of patients does not necessarily mean that the results may be extrapolated to others. Patients going into (and indeed completing) a randomized design are a highly selected population.

A controversial area of HRT is whether *all* women are likely to benefit from the therapy. Detecting women who especially benefit from HRT is a complex medical decision which demands individual counselling based on scientific evidence.

A further integration of biochemical, physiological, clinical and epidemiological findings with special emphasis on differences in the pathogenesis and the pathophysiology of subtypes of cardiovascular diseases, as well as differences in risk profiles, is needed.

References

1. Grodstein F, Stampfer M. The epidemiology of coronary heart disease and estrogen replacement in postmenopausal women. *Prog Cardiovasc Dis* 1995; **38**: 199–210.

2. Matthews KA, Kuller LH, Wing RR *et al.* Prior to use of estrogen replacement therapy, are users healthier than nonusers? *Am J Epidemiol* 1996; **143**: 971–978.

3. Lindenstrøm E, Boysen G, Nyboe J, Appleyard M. Stroke incidence in Copenhagen, 1976–1988. *Stroke* 1992; **23**: 28–32.

4. Grodstein F, Manson JE, Colditz GA *et al.* A prospective observational study of postmenopausal hormone therapy and primary prevention of cardiovascular disease. *Ann Int Med* 2000; **133**: 933–941.

5. Pedersen AT, Lidegaard Ø, Kreiner S, Ottesen B. Hormone replacement therapy and risk of non-fatal stroke. *Lancet* 1997; **350**: 1277–1283.

6. Rosenberg SH, Fausone V, Clark R. The role of estrogens as a risk factor for stroke in postmenopausal women. *West J Med* 1980; **133**: 292–296.

7. Pfeffer RI. Estrogen use, hypertension and stroke in postmenopausal women. *J Chron Dis* 1978; **31**:389–398.

8. Grodstein F, Stampfer MJ, Manson JE *et al.* Postmenopausal estrogen and progestin use and the risk of cardiovascular disease. *N Engl J Med* 1996; **335**: 453–461.

9. Falkeborn M, Persson I, Terent A *et al.* Hormone replacement therapy and the risk of stroke: follow-up of a population-based cohort in Sweden. *Arch Intern Med* 1993; **153**: 1201–1209.

10. Finucane FF, Madans JH, Busch TL, Wolf PH, Kleinman JC. Decreased risk of stroke among postmenopausal hormone users: results from a national cohort. *Arch Intern Med* 1993; **153**: 73–79.

11. Stampfer MJ, Colditz GA, Willett WC *et al.* Postmenopausal estrogen therapy and cardiovascular disease: ten-year follow-up from the Nurses Health Study. *N Engl J Med* 1991; **325**: 756–762.

12. Boysen G, Nyboe J, Appleyard M. Stroke incidence and risk factors for stroke in Copenhagen, Denmark. *Stroke* 1988; **19**: 1345–1353.

13. Hunt K, Vessey M, McPherson K. Mortality in a cohort of long-term users of hormone replacement therapy: an updated analysis. *Br J Obstet Gynaecol* 1990; **97**: 1080–1086.

14. Paganini-Hill A, Ross RK, Henderson BE. Postmenopausal oestrogen treatment and stroke: a prospective study. *BMJ* 1988; **297**: 519–522.

15. Busch TL, Barrett-Connor E, Cowan LD *et al.* Cardiovascular mortality and non-contraceptive use of estrogen in women: results from the Lipid Research Clinics Program Follow-up Study. *Circulation* 1987; **75**: 1102–1109.

16. Daly E, Vessey MP, Hawkins MM *et al.* Risk of venous thromboembolism in users of hormone replacement therapy. *Lancet* 1996; **348**: 977–980.

17. Jick H, Derby LE, Myers MW, Vasilakis C, Newton KM. Risk of hospital admission for idiopathic venous thromboembolism among users of postmenopausal oestrogens. *Lancet* 1996; **348**: 981–983.

18. Grodstein F, Stampfer MJ, Goldhaber SZ *et al.* Prospective study of exogenous hormones and risk of pulmonary embolism in women. *Lancet* 1996; **348**: 983–987.

19. Daly E, Vessey MP, Painter R, Hawkins MM. Case-control study of venous thromboembolism risk in users of hormone replacement therapy. *Lancet* 1996; **348**: 1027.

20. Gutthann SP, Rodriguez LAG, Castellsague J, Oliart AD. Hormone replacement therapy and risk of venous thromboembolism: population based case-control study. *BMJ* 1997; **314**: 796–800.

21. Grady D, Wenger NK, Herrington D *et al.* Postmenopausal hormone therapy increases risk for venous thromboembolic disease. The Heart and Estrogen/Progestin Replacement Study. *Ann Intern Med* 2000; **132**: 689–696.

22. Mendelsohn ME, Karas RH. Mechanisms of disease: the protective effects of estrogen on the cardiovascular system. *N Engl J Med* 1999; **340**: 1801–1811.

Hormone replacement therapy and Alzheimer's disease

Therese van Amelsvoort, Declan Murphy

10

Introduction

There are significant age and sex differences in cognitive ability and brain disease. For example, women generally perform better than men in verbal fluency tests, whereas men perform better on tests of spatial ability. Similarly women suffer more often from depression and Alzheimer's disease (AD), whereas autism is seen more often in men. The biological basis for these gender differences is unknown. However, these observations do suggest that oestrogen and/or the X chromosome may play a role in brain development and ageing. In this chapter we will discuss studies investigating the effects of oestrogen and the X chromosome on normal brain development and ageing, and how they are relevant to Alzheimer's disease.

Gender differences in brain ageing

Ageing of the normal brain is accompanied by changes in brain structure, function, and metabolism; but there are significant gender differences in brain ageing. For example, brain atrophy starts earlier in men;[1] however, once started, atrophy occurs more rapidly in women.[2] In addition, Murphy et al[3] have reported that age-related loss of brain tissue was significantly greater in males than females in the whole brain and frontal and temporal lobes, whereas the loss was greater in females than males in the hippocampus and parietal lobes. A study measuring glucose metabolism and using positron emission tomography (PET) and ^{18}F-2-fluoro-2-deoxy-D-glucose (FDG), showed that the age-related decline in brain metabolism is asymmetric in males, but symmetric in females, and that women have significant age-related decreases in hippocampal glucose metabolism, but men do not.[3] These gender differences occur in regions that are essential to cognitive function and are implicated in neuropsychiatric disorder. They may therefore underlie gender differences in the prevalence and symptomatology of age-related neuropsychiatric disorders, such as AD. For example, women are more likely to develop AD than men, and this cannot be explained solely by their longer life expectancy, since women also have greater disease severity and a higher age-adjusted prevalence of AD than men.

Alzheimer's disease

The prevalence of AD increases dramatically with age—from less than 1% at age 65 to about 15% of people in their eighties.[4] AD is accompanied by progressive cognitive impairment, and this has an enormous impact on the quality of life of patients and their caregivers. Risk factors for AD include a positive family history, presence of Down's syndrome, head injury, female sex, hypothyroidism, depression, and the possession of the apolipoprotein E4 gene. In contrast, education, smoking, and non-steroidal anti-inflammatory agents may be protective factors.[5] On a cellular level, the disease is characterized by neuronal loss, accumulation of intracellular neurofibrillary tangles, and extracellular senile plaques in the hippocampus and association neocortex. Much progress has been made in understanding the aetiology and pathology of AD (including the identification of susceptibility genes). Nevertheless no major success has been gained so far in the treatment of AD.

The search for pharmacological treatments of AD has mainly focused on the major deficits in the cholinergic system, including selective loss of basal forebrain cholinergic neurones, decreased activity of choline acetyltransferase (ChAT)—an enzyme involved in the synthesis of acetylcholine—and decreased activity of acetylcholinesterase (AChE)—an enzyme involved in the breakdown of acetylcholine. Trials with precursors of acetylcholine and cholinesterase inhibitors have demonstrated only limited cognitive improvement, and many have significant unwanted side-effects. Also, the cognitive improvement seen in trials with cholinesterase inhibitors in AD was reported to be most evident in women who were also receiving hormone replacement therapy (HRT).[6] Nevertheless, the first selective cholinesterase inhibitor, donepezil hydrochloride, has now been licensed in the UK as symptomatic treatment for mild to moderate AD. Meanwhile, the search for other possible treatment strategies continues, and more recently scientists have been challenged by the potential therapeutic effects of oestrogens. It is now becoming clear that oestrogens do more than regulate sexual and reproductive behaviour, and that, in addition to their well-known effects on bones and heart, oestrogens have significant effects on brain structure and function.

Oestrogen's actions on brain structure

There is now good evidence that sex steroids (1) directly modulate brain development and ageing,[3,7] (2) directly affect neurochemical systems that are affected in normal ageing as well as in AD and other neuropsychiatric disorders, (3) indirectly decrease cell ageing by antagonizing the effects of oxidants and other neurotoxic compounds in the brain and by assisting nerve growth factors.

Oestrogens increase synaptic and dendritic spine density in the hippocampus—a brain region that is crucial to memory function, and which is significantly affected in AD. For example, in rats following bilateral oophorectomy there is a significant decrease in dendritic spine density in CA1 pyramidal cells. However, this is prevented by administration of oestrogens, and synaptic spine density is significantly related to circulating oestradiol levels.[8]

Previously, it was unclear how these oestrogen-induced dendritic changes affected neuronal function. However, recently it has been demonstrated that oestrogen induces an increase in N-methyl-D-aspartate (NMDA) receptors in rat hippocampal neurons, in the same region where an increase in dendritic spines is found. This is of importance because the NMDA receptor is a membrane protein that detects incoming signals from the excitatory neurotransmitter glutamate. Thus, the 'new' oestrogen-induced spines are now thought to be related to NMDA-type synapses.[9,10]

Oestrogens also directly affect neurochemical transmitter systems affected in normal ageing, AD, and other neuropsychiatric disorders. For example, oestrogens can modulate the serotonergic, cholinergic, and dopaminergic systems. These neurochemical effects of oestrogen may partially explain why depression occurs more often in women, and why AD and very late onset schizophrenia are more common in postmenopausal women, i.e. when levels of circulating oestrogens are low. The oestrogen-induced enhancement of the cholinergic system may be of particular relevance in AD because some of the cognitive impairments in AD are probably secondary to significant cholinergic deficits. Administration of oestrogens to ovariectomized rats increases the activity of ChAT in the basal forebrain, and in two of its projection areas—the CA1 subfield of the hippocampus and the frontal cortex. It is thought that the increased ChAT activity is caused by inducing de novo synthesis of the enzyme in the basal forebrain, with subsequent axonal transport to the CA1 region of the hippocampus and the frontal cortex.[11]

In addition to direct effects on neurons, oestrogens also act with neurotrophins (such as nerve growth factor) to stimulate nerve cell growth indirectly. Receptors for oestrogen and neurotrophins are located on the same neurons in rodent basal forebrain, hippocampus, and cerebral cortex, and this co-localization may be important for the survival of neurons.[12] Oestrogen also has a neuroprotective action[13] against several toxins that boost production of free radicals, including glutamate (which is toxic in high concentrations) and β amyloid. Recently it has been shown that oestrogen can reduce the neuronal generation of β amyloid.[14] Oestrogen may also act as an antioxidant[15]—however, recent findings suggest that the neuroprotective antioxidant activity of oestrogens is dependent on the presence of the hydroxyl group in the C3 position on the A ring of the steroid molecule.[16] Furthermore, Green et al[17] found that the oestrogen molecule also needs a phenolic ring A and at least three rings of the steroid nucleus for its neuroprotective actions. Other indirect beneficial effects of oestrogens on the brain include: (1) prevention of glucocorticoid-induced hippocampal neuronal damage,[18,19] (2) enhancement of cerebral blood flow,[20] and (3) possibly an interaction with apolipoprotein E4, a protein commonly found in AD.[21]

Oestrogen's actions on cognitive function

As noted above, sex steroids are crucial to the development and ageing of the hippocampus and parietal lobe—brain areas significantly affected in AD.[3,7] Moreover, animal studies have demonstrated significant effects of oestrogens on neuronal structures and neurochemical systems affected in AD. But what clinical evidence is there that sex steroids may have a significant role in the genesis and treatment of AD?

Over recent years several studies have looked at the effects of oestrogen on cognitive function in healthy postmenopausal women. The results of these studies have been conflicting, which most likely reflects methodological differences. Some authors have reported beneficial effects of oestrogens on memory function in postmenopausal women.[22,23] Sherwin[24] reported that surgically menopausal (oophorectomized) women have a decrement in cognitive performance postoperatively which is related to a decrease in their plasma levels of circulating sex steroids; subsequent administration of oestrogens improves their scores on cognitive tasks. Jacobs *et al*[25] reported in a longitudinal study that a history of oestrogen use during the postmenopausal period was associated with higher scores on verbal memory, language, and abstract reasoning. Subsequently, over a 2 year follow-up period oestrogen users increased their scores on verbal memory tasks whereas non-users showed a decrease in their scores. Other workers, however, have not found any positive effects of oestrogen on cognitive function in cross-sectional studies in older women.[26] Most studies that report positive effects of oestrogen report improvement in verbal memory. However, often non-verbal tasks were not included in these studies. A recent longitudinal study reported that healthy, postmenopausal women on long-term HRT performed better than postmenopausal women who had never taken HRT on the Benton Visual Retention Test (a test for short-term visual memory, visual perception, and constructional skills).[27] Further support for oestrogen's effects on non-verbal tasks comes

from a recent functional imaging study which demonstrates oestrogen-induced alterations in brain activation patterns during verbal and non-verbal working memory tasks in frontal and parietal regions in postmenopausal women.[28] Thus, there is recent evidence that oestrogen affects not only verbal but also non-verbal aspects of cognitive function in healthy postmenopausal women.

Studies on HRT and AD

Epidemiological studies have reported that the prevalence of AD is significantly decreased in females on HRT, and that women with AD who are taking HRT have significantly milder disease than those who are not.[29] A recent longitudinal study reported that prolonged use of HRT decreases the risk, and delays the onset, of AD; moreover, use of oestrogen for longer than one year reduced the risk of developing AD by 5% annually.[30] These results are promising, and point to the need for further prospective studies of HRT in postmenopausal women with and without AD.

Results of early clinical trials of HRT in people with AD are also promising but require replication. For example, one clinical trial reported that three of seven women with AD improved on measures of attention, orientation, mood, and social interaction after six weeks of low dosages of oestradiol treatment, but the improvement was lost after

oestradiol was discontinued.[31] In another
study, women with AD who were using
oestrogen had significantly better scores on the
Alzheimer's Disease Assessment Scale
(ADAS-Cog, a standard instrument used in
AD clinical trials) than women with AD who
did not take oestrogens.[32]

The X chromosomes

Turner's syndrome provides a biological
model to investigate the effects of the X
chromosome and sex steroids on the brain,
because women with Turner's syndrome (TS;
45,X) normally have only one X chromosome
instead of two, and they do not produce
endogenous oestrogens. However, some
people with TS have a mosaic karyotype
(45,X/46,XX or 45,X/47,XXX).
Neuropsychological studies have shown that
people with TS have better verbal than
visuospatial skills and have abnormalities of
social interaction.[33] A quantitative MRI study
of females with TS reported significant
bilateral decreases in the volume of the
hippocampus, parieto-occipital brain matter,
and lenticular and thalamic nuclei compared
to normal controls (46,XX). Moreover, the
cerebral hemisphere, caudate, and lenticular
and thalamic nuclei showed 'X chromosome
dosage effects', indicating that these structures
depend upon the X chromosome to develop
normally. Hippocampal volume was decreased
in TS subjects, but did not show these 'X

chromosome dosage effects', suggesting that
hippocampal development depends to a
greater degree on sex steroids.[?] Resting brain
glucose metabolism has also been compared in
TS females and controls, using FDG-PET.
Clark et al[34] reported decreased metabolism
in occipital and parietal cortices, and recently
Murphy et al[35] reported that TS was
associated with relative bilateral
hypometabolism in the insula and association
neocortices. In TS females there were also
significant differences in cortical functional
relationships originating bilaterally in the
occipital cortices, and within the right
hemisphere. Also, 'X chromosome dosage'
effects existed in language ability and left
middle temporal lobe metabolism, and in
neuropsychological test scores and asymmetry
of parietal metabolism, indicating that the X
chromosome is involved in the function of the
left and right association neocortices, and that
TS brain metabolic abnormalities are
associated with cognitive deficits. Thus, the X
chromosome and sex steroids appear to have
differential effects on brain structure and
function, and these may explain some of the
neuropsychological and social deficits that are
seen in TS. Recently, a study by Skuse et al[36]
reported that TS females with a paternally
derived X chromosome have better social
skills, higher verbal IQ scores and performed
better on a behavioural inhibition task than
TS females with a maternally derived X
chromosome. Skuse et al suggested that social

functioning is influenced by an imprinted gene on the X chromosome which is switched off when the gene is inherited from the mother.

Conclusions

With the growth in numbers of the older population, it can be expected that AD will become an increasing public health problem. Women are particularly at risk and the role of sex steroids and their effects on the brain have been a major focus in AD research over recent years. There is evidence that sex steroids and X chromosomes modulate brain development and ageing, and can affect cognitive function. Epidemiological, neuropsychological, and biological studies appear to support the hypothesis that oestrogens may be implicated in AD's genesis and treatment. Oestrogens interact with neuronal networks at many different levels, and may affect some of the risk factors for AD. Currently, routine therapeutic use of oestrogens in women with AD is not justified, and more prospective clinical trials are required. In the future new oestrogens may be synthesized which have the neuroprotective characteristics of the currently available oestrogens but which do not carry the same side-effects (e.g. uterine carcinoma). The recent finding that certain subtypes of oestrogens may be more neuroprotective than others may help us to identify such a compound.[16,17] The effect of the new selective oestrogen receptor modulators (SERMs)—which have less side-effects on the breast and endometrium—on the central nervous system is not yet known.[37] In men, the use of such a compound without feminizing effects, or testosterone (which is converted to the oestrogen metabolite oestradiol by intraneuronal aromatization)[38] could be explored.

In conclusion, besides the need for clinical trials in people with AD there is a continuing search for a more selective oestrogen preparation without the unwanted side-effects of current preparations.

References

1. Kaye JA, DeCarli CD, Luxenberg JS *et al.* The significance of age-related enlargement of the cerebral ventricles in healthy men and women measured by quantitative computed X-ray tomography. *J Am Geriatr Soc* 1992; **40**: 225–231.

2. Takeda S, Matsuzawa T. Age-related brain atrophy: a study with computed tomography. *J Gerontol* 1985; **40**: 159–163.

3. Murphy DGM, DeCarli C, McIntosh A *et al.* Sex differences in human brain morphometry and metabolism: an in vivo quantitative magnetic resonance imaging and positron emission tomography study on the effect of aging. *Arch Gen Psychiatry* 1996; **53**: 585–594.

4. Skoog I, Nilsson L, Palmertz B *et al.* A population based study of senile dementia in 85 year olds. *N Engl J Med* 1993; **328**: 153–158.

5. Burns A, Murphy D. Protection against Alzheimer's disease? *Lancet* 1996; **348**: 420–421.

6. Schneider LS, Farlow MR, Henderson VW *et al.* Effects of estrogen replacement therapy on response to tacrine in patients with Alzheimer's disease. *Neurology* 1996; **46**: 1580–1584.

7. Murphy DGM, DeCarli C, Daly E *et al.* X-chromosome effects on female brains: a magnetic resonance imaging study of Turner's syndrome. *Lancet* 1993; **342**: 1197–1200.

8. Gould E, Woolley CS, Frankfurt M *et al.* Gonadal steroids regulate dendritic spine density in hippocampal pyramidal cells in adulthood. *J Neurosci* 1990; **10**: 1286–1291.

9. Gazzaley AH, Weiland NG, McEwen BS *et al.* Differential regulations of NMDAR1 mRNA and protein by estradiol in the rat hippocampus. *J Neurosci* 1996; **16**(21): 6830–6838.

10. Woolley CS, Weiland NG, McEwen BS *et al.* Estradiol increases the sensitivity of hippocampal CA1 pyramidal cells to NMDA receptor-mediated synaptic input: correlation with dendritic spine density. *J Neurosci* 1997; **17**(5): 1848–1859.

11. Luine V. Estradiol increases choline acetyltransferase activity in specific basal forebrain nuclei and projection areas of female rats. *Experimental Neurol* 1985; **89**: 484–490.

12. Toran-Allerand CD. The estrogen/neurotrophin connection during neural development: is co-localization of estrogen receptor with the neurotrophins and their receptors biologically relevant? *Developmental Neurosci* 1996; **18**: 36.

13. Simpkins JW, Singh M, Bishop J. The potential role for estrogen replacement therapy in the treatment of the cognitive decline and neurodegeneration associated with Alzheimer's disease. *Neurobiol Aging* 1994; **15** (suppl 2): S195–197.

14. Xu H, Guoras GK, Greenfield JP *et al.* Oestrogen reduces neuronal generation of Alzheimer β amyloid peptides. *Nature Med* 1998; **4**(4): 447–451.

15. Behl C, Widmann, Trapp T, Holsboer F. 17-Beta oestradiol protects neurons from oxidative stress-induced cell death in vitro. *Biochem Biophys Res Commun* 1995; **216**: 473–482.

16. Behl C, Skutella T, Lezoualc'h F *et al.* Neuroprotection against oxidative stress by estrogens: structure–activity relationship. *Molecular Pharmacol* 1997; **51**: 535–541.

17. Green PS, Gordon K, Simpkins JW. Phenolic ring requirement for the neuroprotective effects of steroids. *J Steroid Biochem Mol Biol* 1997; **63**(4–6): 229–235.

18. Mizoguchi K, Tatsuhide T, De-Hua C *et al.* Stress-induced neuronal death in the hippocampus of castrated rats. *Neurosci Lett* 1992; **138**: 157–160.

19. Sapolsky RM, Plotsky PM. Hypercortisolism and its possible neural bases. *Biol Psychiatry* 1990; **27**: 937–952.

20. Ohkura T, Isse K, Akazawa K *et al.* Evaluation of estrogen treatment in female patients with dementia of the Alzheimer type. *Endocrine J* 1994; **41**(4): 361–371.

21. Honjo H, Tanaka K, Kashiwagi T *et al.* Senile dementia—Alzheimer's type and estrogen. *Hormone Metab Res* 1995; **27**: 204–207.

22. Robinson D, Friedman L, Marcus R *et al.* Estrogen replacement therapy and memory in older women. *J Am Geriatr Soc* 1994; **42**: 919–922.

23. Kimura D. Estrogen replacement therapy may protect against intellectual decline in post menopausal women. *Hormones & Behaviour* 1995; **29**: 312–321.

24. Sherwin BB. Estrogen and/or androgen replacement therapy and cognitive functioning in surgically menopausal women. *Psychoneuroendocrinology* 1988; **13**(4): 345–357.

25. Jacobs DM, Tang MX, Stern Y *et al.* Cognitive function in nondemented older women who took estrogen after menopause. *Neurology* 1998; **50**: 368–373.

26. Barret-Connor E, Silverstein D. Estrogen replacement therapy and cognitive function in older women. *JAMA* 1993; **269**: 2637–2641.

27. Resnick SM, Metter EJ, Zondermann AB. Estrogen replacement therapy and longitudinal decline in visual memory: a possible protective effect? *Neurology* 1997; **49**: 1491–1497.

28. Shaywitz E, Shaywitz BA, Pugh KR *et al.* Effect of estrogen on brain activation patterns in postmenopausal women during working memory tasks. *JAMA* 1999; **281**: 1197–1202.

29. Henderson V, Paganini-Hill A, Emanuel C *et al.* Estrogen replacement therapy in older women. *Arch Neurol* 1994; **51**: 896–900.

30. Tang M, Jacobs D, Stern Y *et al.* Effects of oestrogen during menopause on risk and age at onset of Alzheimer's disease. *Lancet* 1996; **348**: 429–432.

31. Fillit H, Weinreb H, Cholst I *et al.* Observations in a preliminary open trial of estradiol therapy for senile dementia-Alzheimer's type. *Psychoneuroendocrinology* 1986; **11**: 337–345.

32. Doraismay PM, Krishen A, Martin WL *et al.* Gender, concurrent oestrogen use and cognition in Alzheimer's disease. *Int J Geriatr Psychopharmacol* 1997; **40**: 34–37.

33. Murphy DGM, Allen G, Haxby JV *et al.* The effects of sex steroids, and the X chromosome, on female brain function: a study of the neuropsychology of adult Turner syndrome. *Neuropsychologia* 1994; **32**(11): 1309–1323.

34. Clark C, Klonoff H, Hayden M. Regional cerebral glucose metabolism in Turner syndrome. *Can J Neurol Sci* 1990; **17**: 140–144.

35. Murphy DGM, Mentis MJ, Pietrini P *et al.* A PET study Turner's syndrome: effects of sex steroids and the X chromosome on the brain. *Biol Psychiatry* 1997; **41**: 285–298.

36. Skuse DH, James RS, Bishop DVM *et al.* Evidence from Turner's syndrome of an imprinted X-linked locus affecting cognitive function. *Nature* 1997; **387**: 705–708.

37. Beardsworth SA, Purdie DW, Kearney CE. Selective oestrogen receptor modulation: an alternative to conventional oestrogen. *Curr Obstet Gynaecol* 1998; **8**(2): 96–101.

38. MacLusky NJ, Naftolin F. Sexual differentiation of the central nervous system. *Science* 1981; **211**: 1294–1303.

Hormone replacement therapy and the breast

Jo Marsden

11

Introduction

One hundred years ago, George Beatson described partial clinical responses in three premenopausal women with advanced breast cancer following surgical oophorectomy.[1] His conclusion that 'we must look . . . to the ovaries as the seat of the exciting cause of (breast) cancer' laid the foundations for the current understanding of the oestrogen sensitivity of this disease and the concept underlying endocrine breast cancer therapy that tumours are deprived of oestrogen derived from the plasma or synthesized locally in breast tissue itself.

Epidemiological, in vitro and in vivo experimental evidence has since confirmed the role of endogenous oestrogens in the promotion of breast cancer cell growth[2,3] and recent prospective observational studies have shown significant associations between elevations in circulating serum oestradiol and its metabolites and the risk of developing postmenopausal breast cancer or breast cancer recurrence.[4–9] Ovarian ablation and tamoxifen (a mixed oestrogen agonist and antagonist) have been shown to improve significantly the disease-free and overall survival of women with oestrogen receptor (ER) positive breast cancer;[10,11] the more widespread use of adjuvant therapy is considered to account for the significant (10%) reduction in breast cancer mortality in England and Wales observed between 1985 and 1995.[12] Attention has, furthermore, been focused on the link between oestrogens and breast cancer, given that tamoxifen and the selective oestrogen receptor modulator (SERM) raloxifene have both been associated with a decrease in the incidence of ER-positive breast cancer.[13,14]

The benefits of hormone replacement therapy (HRT) in relieving oestrogen deficiency symptoms and in the longer term conferring protection against osteoporosis and probably the primary prevention of arterial disease are recognized. Despite these obvious benefits the overwhelming evidence for the oestrogen dependency of breast cancer implies that HRT exposure will increase the risk of developing breast cancer and disease recurrence. However, review of available clinical data suggests that this may not be the cause and demonstrates that breast cancer is a disease that defies theoretical predictions.

Indirect evidence that HRT may not stimulate the growth of breast cancer cells

Although endocrine therapy has an established role in the treatment of breast cancer, our understanding of the basic mechanisms responsible for the efficacy of such treatment is incomplete given the observation that mean oestradiol levels in breast tumours from premenopausal and postmenopausal women do not differ significantly despite a 10-fold difference in respective circulating oestradiol levels.[15] Tamoxifen is an effective treatment in premenopausal women with ER-positive disease even though it induces a hyperoestrogenic state, in which serum oestradiol levels can exceed those observed during the peak of the follicular phase of the menstrual cycle by 2–3-fold.[11,16]

The assumption that oestrogens alone are responsible for the development and progression of breast cancer can be questioned further in view of the paradoxical behaviour of breast cancer when exposed to high serum levels of exogenous or endogenous oestrogen, where prognosis does not appear to be adversely affected. For example, pharmacological doses of oestrogens were used in the palliation of postmenopausal women with advanced breast cancer before the advent of tamoxifen,[17] and in randomized adjuvant breast cancer trials diethylstilbestrol has been shown to have an equivalent disease-free and overall survival benefit compared with tamoxifen in postmenopausal women, irrespective of tumour ER status.[18] There is also some evidence that the prognosis for breast cancer patients who become pregnant after a diagnosis of breast cancer may be improved, although the possibility that those becoming pregnant were a self-selected, good prognosis group at low risk of recurrence cannot be excluded. In a series of 227 patients aged under 35 years at diagnosis who received chemotherapy, lower rates of recurrence and death were reported in 25 women who subsequently became pregnant.[19] Von Scholtz et al[20] compared 50 women becoming pregnant after diagnosis with a control group of 2000 women. The hazard ratio, after adjustment for nodal status and age, was 0.48 (95% confidence interval 0.02–1.29) for the group who became pregnant. In isolation, none of these arguments can be used as evidence that HRT will not influence breast cancer risk. They do, however, reinforce the view that the aetiology of this disease is complex and poorly understood.

Does oestrogen replacement therapy increase the risk of developing breast cancer?

Recent prospective observational studies have shown a significant association between the risk of developing postmenopausal breast cancer and increases in circulating serum oestrogens. This increase in risk, however, occurs with very small increments in serum oestrogens, none of which exceed the upper limit of the normal postmenopausal range, i.e. <100 pmol/l.[4–9] Collectively, these studies suggest that exposure to oral, transdermal, or low dose implant (i.e. 25 µg oestradiol) replacement therapy that results in a mean range of serum oestradiol of 200–360 pmol/l

will increase the risk of developing postmenopausal breast cancer. However, if the risk of developing breast cancer were related simply to levels of circulating oestrogens, it is surprising that the numerous clinical studies undertaken to evaluate the effect of HRT on the risk of this disease have produced contradictory findings. Since all these studies have been case–control or cohort in design and therefore lacked appropriate randomized controlled groups for comparison, they are open to the influence of bias in patient selection, recall, surveillance, and interview techniques. Increased mammographic surveillance, for example, could explain the increase in the reported incidence of ductal carcinoma in situ in HRT compared with non-HRT users.[21] To allow for the effect of systematic errors, confounders, and biases, it has been recommended that individual epidemiological studies should not be considered persuasive of an association unless the lower limit of the calculated 95% confidence interval falls at least above a threefold risk.[22] No single study investigating the association between HRT and breast cancer risk has reported an increase in risk of that magnitude.

Only one placebo-controlled, randomized trial of HRT has been completed in which breast cancer was a primary end-point. Here, a sequential preparation was prescribed (i.e. conjugated oestrogens 2.5 mg/day and medroxyprogesterone acetate 10 mg/day) and was not shown to have any significant effect on the risk of developing breast cancer. Despite the long follow-up of 22 years, however, patient numbers were far too small for these results to be considered conclusive.[23]

In an attempt to clarify this controversy, several meta-analyses have been undertaken (*Table 11.1*).[24–29] Overall, these suggest that current long-term use of HRT (i.e. > 10 years) is associated with a slight increase in the risk of developing breast cancer (range of relative risk 1.2–1.3). The most recently published re-analysis of 51 individual studies, worldwide,[30] calculated that for every year that HRT is used it increases the relative risk of developing breast cancer by 1.023 (95% confidence interval 1.011–1.036) and that with more than 5 years' use (although the median duration use of HRT in this subgroup of women was in fact 11 years) the relative lifetime risk of developing breast cancer is 1.35 (95% confidence interval 1.21–1.49). Based on these calculations, it has been estimated that if HRT is commenced at the age of 50 years, 5 years' continuous use will be associated with two extra breast cancers, 10 years' use with six extra breast cancers, and 15 years use with 12 extra cancers per 1000 women. A similar pattern of risk with the use of HRT was also calculated for women with a family history of breast carcinoma, but the 99% confidence intervals were very wide and encompassed unity. Failure of investigators in individual trials to accurately document

family history renders it impossible to determine whether women investigated were truly at an increased risk of breast cancer or not. Tumours developing in women at high risk of breast cancer owing to inherited mutations in the BRCA1 and BRCA2 genes, which account for 75% of familial disease, may have a hormone resistant phenotype in that they are usually high grade, ER and progesterone receptor (PgR) negative and therefore resistant to tamoxifen therapy.[31] Reproductive factors, however, do appear to be important in the development of these tumours. Rebbeck *et al*[32] reported a significant decrease in the incidence of breast cancer in women with BRCA1 mutations who underwent bilateral oophorectomy for the prophylaxis of ovarian cancer. However, the use of 'add-back' HRT by some women to prevent the unwanted effects of premature oestrogen deficiency did not appear to negate the benefit of oophorectomy for breast cancer risk. The collaborative re-analysis did not examine the role of HRT in women at high risk of developing breast cancer due to benign breast disease, which encompasses a range of conditions of the breast, of which only atypical ductal or lobular hyperplasia are associated with a significant 3–4-fold increase in the risk of developing breast cancer. Most studies have not categorized benign breast disease and therefore it is very difficult to interpret the available data. In their meta-analysis, Dupont and Page[25] concluded that

Table 11.1
Meta-analyses of HRT and breast cancer risk.

Reference	No of studies	Any HRT use RR (95% CI)	Duration of use RR (95% CI)
24	Not stated	1.01 (0.95–1.08)	
25	28	1.07 (1.00–1.05)	
26	16	1.0	1.30 (1.20–1.60) > 15 years
27	10	1.0	1.23 (1.04–1.51) ≥ 10 years
28	37 Combined HRT (n = 3 studies)	1.06 (1.00–1.12) 0.99 (0.72–1.36) ever use	1.20 (no CI) ≥8 years
29	31 Combined HRT (n = 4 studies)	1.40 (1.20–1.63) current use 1.13 (0.78–1.64) ever use	1.23 (1.08–1.40) > 10 years
30	51 Combined HRT (n not stated)		1.35 (1.21–1.49) > 5 years 1.53 (SE 0.33) ≥ 5 years

RR = relative risk; CI = confidence interval; SE = standard error.

there was no definitive evidence to support the contra-indication of HRT in women with a history of benign breast disease. This is further supported by their retrospective cohort study, in which accurate categorization of benign breast disease was made.[33]

Combined HRT and breast cancer risk

The role of progestins in the aetiology of breast cancer remains to be clarified. It has been hypothesized that progestins will confer protection against the development of breast cancer or breast cancer recurrence. This is based on the observations that the relative risk of developing breast cancer is increased fivefold in women with luteal phase progesterone deficiency[34] and that the survival of premenopausal women with early stage breast cancer may be increased if they are operated on during the luteal phase of the menstrual cycle.[35] Alternatively, it has been postulated that progestins may increase the risk of developing breast cancer, since most proliferative breast activity occurs during the luteal phase of the menstrual cycle, when both oestrogen and progesterone levels are elevated.[36] Complicating matters further is the fact that it is not known whether the class of progestin prescribed or the pattern of progestin prescription (i.e. continuous or combined) is relevant in this context.

Theoretical arguments favour the avoidance of the 19-nortestosterone derivatives, since, compared with the C21 progesterone derivatives, the former exhibit relatively greater androgenic and oestrogenic properties. However, the 19-nortestosterone derivative lynestrenol significantly reduces the ER content of cellular aspirates from women with benign breast disease, suggesting an inhibition of oestrogen stimulation of breast epithelial cells in vivo.[37] Furthermore, breast cancer risk has not been reported to be increased in women treated solely with this class of progestin for benign breast disease (relative risk 0.48, 95% confidence interval 0.25–0.90).[38]

The hypothesis that continuous combined, rather than sequential HRT will confer protection against the development of breast cancer is based on in vitro data in which the continuous application of progestins with oestrogens induces a sustained inhibitory effect on oestrogen-driven cell replication.[39] This inhibitory response appears to be mediated via a variety of cellular pathways, including an increase in the enzymatic conversion of oestradiol to oestrone sulphate, promotion of apoptosis, inhibition of the proto-oncogenes c-myc and c-fos, and a decrease in the breast cancer growth factor cathepsin D.[40] As progestins down-regulate cellular progesterone receptor (PgR) content, continuous application of unopposed progestin will attenuate this inhibitory effect.

The collaborative re-analysis reported that current long-term use of combined HRT might confer a greater lifetime risk of developing breast cancer than would oestrogen alone.[30] However, the number of breast cancer cases upon which this risk estimate was based was too small for this finding to be considered definitive. Subsequent to this, five observational studies have been published which are all consistent in demonstrating an association between long-term exposure to combined HRT and an increase in the risk of developing breast cancer.[41–45] Unfortunately, since the individual data are expressed in different ways, it is impossible to determine whether this risk is equivalent to that for unopposed oestrogen, or of a greater magnitude. Risk has been reported to be increased with the use of cyclic rather than continuous administration of C21 progesterone derivatives[44,45] but the converse has been reported with the 19 non-testosterone-derived progestins.[43] The small numbers in these subgroup analyses prevent any firm recommendations from being made.

Since most women prescribed HRT have not had a hysterectomy, this is obviously an area that warrants further evaluation.

HRT, breast density, and mammography

Subset analysis of the placebo-controlled, randomized Postmenopausal Estrogen/Progestin Interventions (PEPI) Trial has confirmed findings of numerous observational studies reporting an increase in mammographic breast density with exposure to postmenopausal HRT.[46] The results from the PEPI Trial furthermore suggest that mammographic density is increased to a greater degree in women prescribed combined HRT preparations. After 12 months, density increased by 3.5% (95% confidence interval 1.0–12.0%) in women treated with conjugated equine oestrogen (CEE) alone compared with increases of 19.4% (95% confidence interval 9.9–28.9%) and 23.5% (95% confidence interval 11.9–35.1%) in women prescribed CEE plus continuous

medroxyprogesterone or CEE plus cyclic medroxyprogesterone, respectively. It is worth noting, however, that the 95% confidence intervals were wide, particularly for the use of combined therapy.

Although increased breast density is associated with an increase in the risk of developing breast cancer (>75% breast density, relative risk for developing breast cancer 4.35, 95% confidence interval 3.1–6.1)[47] and the use of postmenopausal unopposed or combined HRT is associated with an increase in breast epithelial density,[48] whether either can be used as an accurate surrogate measure for the risk of developing breast cancer or breast cancer recurrence in women taking HRT is unresolved. HRT does appear to reduce the sensitivity and specificity of mammography[49] but it has been reported that cessation of HRT for as little as 2 weeks before mammography could be sufficient to overcome this screening problem.[50]

The Million Women Study, a survey of HRT use in women attending for mammographic breast cancer screening in the United Kingdom, will not provide definitive data about breast cancer risk in the absence of a randomized control group for comparison (Institute of Cancer Research, Epidemiology Unit/NHS Breast Screening Programme). There is no evidence that healthy women on HRT require more frequent mammograms than are received through the National NHS Breast Cancer Screening Programme.[57]

The influence of HRT on breast tumour biology

The recent collaborative re-analysis demonstrated that the small increase in the risk of developing breast cancer associated with HRT exposure disappears completely within 5 years of it being stopped.[27] In conjunction with case reports of breast tumour regression following withdrawal of HRT,[40,41] this suggests that HRT promotes the growth of pre-existing breast cancers rather than initiating carcinogenic change in the breast. There is no evidence at present, however, to suggest that HRT stimulates exclusively the growth of ER-positive disease.

Evidence of the effect of HRT on breast tumour biology and extrapolation to clinical events is unclear. Most studies are flawed in that HRT was not taken up to the day of breast biopsy. It has been shown quite clearly in studies of preoperative hormonal manipulation of primary breast cancers that significant changes in breast tumour receptor status and proliferation rates (i.e. Ki67) can occur after periods as short as 1 week.[54] HRT (both unopposed and combined preparations) was administered up to the day of biopsy in the study of Hargreaves *et al*[55] and shown to induce breast tissue PgR content. However, the lack of any expected associated increase of breast cell proliferation is probably explained by the methodology used, which precludes exclusion of a significant effect on the latter.

In contrast, percutaneous administration of progestin has been shown to inhibit oestrogen-induced breast epithelial cell proliferation.[56] Although assessment of cellular proliferation was more robust in this latter study, the application of percutaneous oestrogen and progestin was via the breast, which results in a significant increment in breast oestradiol levels. As such a difference in breast oestradiol levels has not been seen in comparisons between premenopausal and postmenopausal women, this suggests that administration through the breast is the significant issue but it cannot be related directly to conventional HRT.

The identification of two distinct subtypes of the ER, ERα and ERβ, in the rat, mouse, and human has resulted in a revaluation of the molecular basis for oestrogen activity. At present, the significance of their different tissue distributions and ligand selectivities is unknown and requires further extensive study. How this will influence our understanding of the effect of HRT on breast cell proliferation remains to be answered.

The effect of HRT on breast cancer mortality

With the exception of findings from the Nurses Health Study,[57] use of HRT before a diagnosis of breast cancer does not appear to have an adverse effect on cause-specific or overall mortality (*Table 11.2*).[56–70] Breast

Table 11.2
Mortality in breast cancer patients with a history of previous HRT exposure at time of breast cancer diagnosis.

Reference	Cancer mortality RR (95% CI)	Breast cancer mortality RR (95% CI)
58		0.53, p < 0.007 (CI not stated)
59	0.22 (no CI)	0.73 (0.44–1.22)
60		0.68 (0.52–0.87)
61	0.70 (0.55–0.85)	0.76 (0.45–1.06)
62	0.80 (NS)	0.81, p > 0.05 (CI not stated)
63		No reduction (p > 0.01)
57	0.71 (0.62–0.81) current use 1.04 (0.90–1.13) past use	0.76 (0.56–1.02) current use 0.83 (0.63–1.09) past use
64		0.75 (0.48–1.17) use < 5 years 0.79 (0.83–1.67) use > 5 years
65		0.2 (0.1–0.3) use < 5 years 0.7 (0.5–0.9) use 5–9 years 0.7 (0.5–0.9) use ≥ 10 years
66		0.84 (0.75–0.94) 0.59 (0.40–0.87) natural menopause 0.76 (0.54–1.09) surgical menopause
67		0.92 (0.55–1.54) family history of breast cancer
68		HRT 92% v no HRT 86% (p = 0.07)
69		0.78 (0.63–0.96) use < 5 years 0.77 (0.56–1.08) use ≥ 5 years
70		0.5 (0.3–0.8) current use at diagnosis 2.2 (0.9–5.2) > 144 months after diagnosis

RR = relative risk; CI = confidence interval; NS = non significant.
* Long-term mortality increased in long-term HRT users (i.e. > 10 years), primarily due to increased breast cancer mortality.

tumours diagnosed in women with a history of current or past use of HRT tend to be less clinically advanced in that they are smaller in size and better differentiated but, although some investigators have found a predominance of lymph node negative disease in women exposed to HRT, others have not.[27] Gapstur *et al*[71] observed that HRT use is associated with an increase in the incidence of invasive breast cancer with a favourable histology (i.e. tubular and papillary cancers) but not with the more common invasive ductal or lobular carcinomas, which have a worse overall outcome. The beneficial effect of HRT on subsequent breast cancer mortality seems to occur irrespective of tumour hormone receptor or axillary lymph node status.[68,69] Although prior use of HRT has been reported to be associated with a small increase in the incidence of ipsilateral breast cancer recurrence, the incidence of distant metastatic disease is significantly reduced and mortality is unaffected.[68]

This apparent favourable effect of HRT could be influenced by surveillance bias, in that women requesting HRT tend to have more of an interest in general disease prevention activities such as breast cancer surveillance, or that women with breast cancer are not generally prescribed HRT and will be among the non-users in observational studies. However, these mortality studies suggest that, even if HRT increases the incidence of breast cancer or promotes disease recurrence, it may

not have a detrimental effect on breast cancer versus all-cause mortality, which is the important end-point.

The use of HRT in women previously treated for breast cancer

The management of oestrogen deficiency symptoms in women with breast cancer is becoming an important part of their care, since many experience iatrogenic symptoms induced by their breast cancer therapy. These can include the anti-oestrogenic effects of tamoxifen, chemotherapy-induced ovarian suppression and chemical castration with gonadotrophin-releasing hormone agonists (GnRHa). Cross-sectional studies have demonstrated that at any one time oestrogen deficiency symptoms are the most common adverse effect of adjuvant therapy, occurring in up to 66% of patients aged less than 65 years, and that such symptoms are more bothersome and persist for longer in postmenopausal breast cancer survivors than in healthy postmenopausal women.[72] It is anticipated that the prevalence of treatment-induced oestrogen-deficiency symptoms and the induction of a premature menopause are likely to increase with the more widespread use of adjuvant therapy following the clear survival benefits shown in the most recent worldwide overviews of early breast cancer therapy.[10,11] In addition to the development of hot flushes and night sweats, loss of sexual interest is a frequently reported symptom accompanying endocrine breast cancer therapy.[73] Chemical castration with chemotherapy and GHRHa can produce vaginal dryness, which, along with decreased emotional well-being, is an important predictor of sexual health in breast cancer survivors.[74] Although vaginal dryness and dyspareunia are less frequent in women taking tamoxifen, problems with sexual interest, arousal and orgasm are reported with its use.[75,76]

Concern that HRT may increase the risk of developing recurrent breast cancer has led to considerable interest in the use of alternative therapies for the control of oestrogen-deficiency-related health problems in breast cancer survivors. As treatment options for the prevention of the long-term sequelae of oestrogen deficiency are to be discussed in detail by other authors in this volume, only alternatives for symptom management will be discussed here.

Alternatives to HRT for symptom control have either not been evaluated in controlled prospective studies at all (i.e. all complementary therapies), or have not been shown to have any more than a placebo effect (i.e. evening primrose oil, vitamin E, clonidine, soy phyto-oestrogens).[77–80] There have been anecdotal reports that serotonin-uptake inhibitors reduce hot flushes in breast cancer patients by 50% but there are no controlled clinical data to support this.[81] Low-dose, slow-release topical oestrogen preparations are effective in the alleviation of distressing vaginal symptoms. Since they do not appear to be associated with any significant absorption across the vaginal epithelium, they probably do not exert any oestrogenic effect on the breast, but this requires confirmation.

Low-dose progestins and the synthetic gonadomimetic agent, tibolone, which has weak oestrogen-like, progestogen-like, and androgen-like activity, are hormonal preparations that are being prescribed increasingly to breast cancer patients as safe alternatives to HRT. However, there is a complete lack of any controlled data on their safety and efficacy in breast cancer survivors. Although low-dose progestins have been shown to provide effective symptom relief in the short term (i.e. for 3 months), uncontrolled follow-up of 18 of the original breast cancer patients participating in this study for 3 years found that nearly 40% were still symptomatic on treatment and that troublesome side-effects, which included vaginal bleeding and depressive mood, were common.[82] Tibolone (2.5 mg) appears to be as efficacious as standard dosages of HRT for the control of vasomotor symptoms[83] but there are no data on its use in women with breast cancer. Despite the hypothesis that tibolone may protect against breast cancer recurrence, since it inhibits the conversion of oestrone sulphate to oestradiol in MCF-7 and T-47D breast cancer cell lines,[84] its relative oestrogenic and androgenic activities are reported to increase with the higher dosages that are sometimes required for symptom control, particularly in prematurely menopausal women.[85]

Given the lack of a causal relationship between HRT and breast cancer risk and the known benefits of HRT in relieving menopausal symptoms, HRT has increasingly been prescribed to individual breast cancer patients. Published data from a small number of observational trials of HRT in breast cancer survivors with both early and advanced stage disease have, to date, not demonstrated any increase in disease progression or death from breast cancer, suggesting that HRT may not adversely affect prognosis, even in those women whose tumours were ER-positive (*Table 11.3*).[86–97] Although the ideal frequency for mammographic follow-up of women with breast cancer is not established and current practice is variable, there is no evidence to support such follow-up being performed more often than annually if patients are taking HRT.

In the absence of data from randomized trials, reliable statements about the safety of HRT in this clinical context cannot be made. A pilot study undertaken to ascertain the feasibility of conducting a national randomized trial of HRT in symptomatic women with early stage breast cancer demonstrated high accrual (40%) and compliance (>80%) rates despite detailed, informed consent.[98] This pilot study demonstrated that oestrogen-deficiency symptoms had a significant negative impact on patients' quality of life. Three of the 100 women recruited into this study have developed recurrent breast cancer to date. Two were taking HRT; one was randomized to receive opposed HRT 38 months after diagnosis and developed recurrence after taking HRT for 2 years. The second patient received unopposed HRT 9 years after diagnosis and developed recurrent disease after six weeks' treatment.

Following the successful implementation of this pilot study and patient feedback, which revealed that the management of oestrogen-deficiency symptoms is considered by breast cancer patients to be an important aspect of their care, a large randomized trial of HRT has now been planned in the United Kingdom, and two smaller randomized trials have been established in Sweden. The United Kingdom trial aims to recruit a total of 3000 symptomatic women with stage I or stage II breast cancer, who will be randomized to HRT for two years. It is anticipated that, in addition to providing reliable data on the effects of HRT use on disease-free and overall survival, the question of potential antagonism between HRT and tamoxifen will be answered (*Figure 11.1*).

Table 11.3
HRT after breast cancer—observational studies.

Reference	No of patients	Stage of disease	Type of HRT	Median time from diagnosis in months (range)	Median duration of use in months (range)	Median follow-up in months (range)	New cancer /recurrence No	%
86	Unknown	I–II	O + Pc	Not stated	3–6	≥ 24 months	0	0
87	25	I–IV	Not stated	26 (0–180)*	35.2 (6–78)*	Not stated	3	12
88	77	I–IV	O and O + Ps	24 (0–324)	27 (1–233)	59 (10–425)	7	9.1
89	35	I–IV	O and O + Ps	31 (0–215)	14.6 (1–44)	43	2	5.7
90	90	I–II	P, O + Ps, and O + Pc	60 (0–300)	18 (3–144)	84 (4–360)	7	7.8
91	43	I–II	Not stated	84 (0–286)	31 (24–142)	144 (46–342)	1	2.3
92	67	Unknown	O	Not known	94 (1–154)	94 (1–454)	0	0
93	61	I–III	O and O + P	44.4 (0–232.8)*	26.4 (0.48–198)*	Not stated	6	9.8
94	189	I–III	Not stated	59 (2–392)	41+ (1–76+)	Not stated	12	6.3
95	120	I–IV	O and O + P	96 (18.24–266.4)	28.8+ (12–127.2)	Not stated	5	4.2

O = unopposed oestrogen; P = unopposed progestin; O + Ps = sequential HRT; O + P = continuous combined HRT; O + Pc = type of combined HRT prescribed not stated.
* Values are means with their respective ranges.

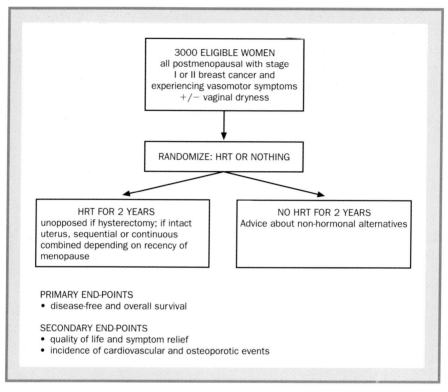

Figure 11.1
The National Randomised Trial of HRT in Symptomatic Women with Early Stage Breast Cancer.

Tamoxifen and HRT— antagonistic or synergistic?

Re-evaluation of the therapeutic role of HRT in breast cancer survivors necessitates consideration of the combined, systemic effects of tamoxifen and HRT, particularly on breast cancer cell proliferation. Concern that HRT may antagonize the anti-neoplastic effect of tamoxifen in breast cancer survivors has not been evaluated in controlled trials and therefore the only evidence available upon which to base any clinical recommendations is that from the tamoxifen chemoprevention trials.

Following the observation of a 50%

reduction in the incidence of contralateral breast cancer in women treated with adjuvant tamoxifen therapy, three randomized tamoxifen chemoprevention trials in women at high risk of developing breast cancer were initiated in the United States, Italy, and the United Kingdom. The largest of these, the National Surgical Adjuvant Breast and Bowel Project P-1 Study (NSABP P-1), reported a 69% reduction in the incidence of ER-positive invasive breast cancer (relative risk 0.31; 95% confidence interval 0.22–0.45) but no difference in the occurrence of ER-negative disease and a 50% reduction in the incidence of non-invasive breast cancer ($p < 0.002$) after a median follow-up of 4.5 years.[12] As a result this trial was stopped prematurely and women taking placebo were given the opportunity to commence tamoxifen. In the absence of any long-term mortality data, however, it is not possible to determine whether this reported benefit of tamoxifen reflects treatment of subclinical disease or a true reduction in the risk of developing breast cancer.

Interim analyses of the Italian and United Kingdom trials have not shown tamoxifen to reduce breast cancer risk.[99,100] Although it has been argued that these smaller trials are not powerful enough to detect any true difference, the fact that the use of HRT was permitted in these trials, and not the NSABP P-1 trial, has been offered as an explanation of the opposing results. HRT, however, did not appear to exert an adverse effect on breast cancer

incidence in the 42% of women taking it during the Royal Marsden Hospital trial but the Italian study reported that tamoxifen reduced the incidence of breast cancer in the 14% of women who received HRT (hazard ratio 0.13; 95% confidence interval 0.02–1.02). Since the European trials have not completed follow-up and the use of HRT in this context was not a primary hypothesis, and nor was its allocation randomized, these preliminary results should be treated with caution and no definitive conclusions should be drawn.

Tamoxifen has a diverse range of clinical effects owing to its complex endocrinological profile. Anti-oestrogenic, partial oestrogen-agonist, and oestrogen-independent activities have all been described and evidence is accumulating that the level of circulating endogenous oestrogen influences the biological activity of tamoxifen. In postmenopausal women, tamoxifen exerts predominantly oestrogenic effects on bone mineral density, serum low density lipoprotein (LDL) cholesterol levels, vaginal epithelium, and the endometrium, where it is associated with a 2–3-fold increase in the risk of developing endometrial cancer. In premenopausal women, however, tamoxifen appears to behave as an anti-oestrogen in that it promotes bone demineralization, has no significant effect on serum cholesterol levels, and may not induce vaginal epithelial cell maturation or endometrial proliferation.[11,101,102]

Preliminary data from the tamoxifen chemoprevention studies suggest that tamoxifen and HRT have a cumulative beneficial effect on femoral bone mineral density, with an annual reported increase of 4%.[101] In contrast, animal studies have shown that the bone-sparing effect of tibolone is prevented by anti-oestrogens.[103] Reports that the oestrogenic effect of tamoxifen on the endometrium is inversely correlated with age suggest that the oestrogen component of combined HRT may protect postmenopausal women against the development of tamoxifen-induced endometrial pathology. Using changes in serum lipoprotein levels as a surrogate for arterial disease events, there does not appear to be any additional benefit of adding HRT to tamoxifen.[101,104]

The selective oestrogen receptor modulator (SERM) raloxifene, which is an analogue of tamoxifen, has been reported to reduce significantly the incidence of postmenopausal ER-positive breast cancer in a meta-analysis of nine randomized, placebo-controlled trials (relative risk 0.46; 95% confidence interval 0.28–0.75).[14] The most recent data from the ongoing Multiple Outcomes of Raloxifene Evaluation (MORE) study have indicated a relative risk of developing breast cancer of 0.35 (95% confidence interval 0.21–0.58) with a median follow-up of 40 months.[105] However, these results should be treated with caution, since osteoporosis prevention and not breast cancer incidence or survival was the primary end point of these trials. A breast cancer chemoprevention trial comparing tamoxifen and raloxifene is planned in the United States, in which breast cancer incidence and mortality will be the main outcome measures. In common with tamoxifen and other SERMs under development, raloxifene is ineffective in treating oestrogen deficiency symptoms and may even induce them and therefore has no role in the treatment of vasomotor symptoms in breast cancer patients. No clinical data exist for cases in which raloxifene and HRT have been prescribed together.

Conclusion

Endogenous oestrogens are implicated in the aetiology of breast cancer, but the role of exogenous hormones remains unclear. Theoretical predictions that HRT will increase breast cancer risk and disease progression have not been substantiated by observational data but it is probable that HRT promotes the growth of pre-existing breast cancers rather than increasing the incidence of the disease per se. This growth promotion, however, does not appear to be associated with an increase in breast cancer mortality and may reflect a selective biological effect on the growth of less aggressive tumours. Two large randomized trials of HRT in healthy women are now

underway in the United States (the
Women's Health Initiative, which was set
up by the National Institutes of Health)
and the United Kingdom (the MRC
WISDOM study; the Women's International
Study of Long-Duration Oestrogen use
after the Menopause). In conjunction with
planned randomized trials in breast cancer
survivors, it is hoped that, ultimately, more
reliable data on the long-term benefits and
risks of HRT will be provided. Until such
data are available, clinicians must rely on
the findings of observational studies, but
in this it is essential that the limitations
incurred by designs of such studies are
appreciated.

References

1. Beatson GT. On the treatment of inoperable
carcinoma of the mamma: suggestions for a
new method of treatment, with illustrative
cases. *Lancet* 1896; **2**: 104–107.

2. Hulka BA, Stark AT. Breast cancer: cause and
prevention. *Lancet* 1995; **346**: 883–887.

3. Howell A, Clarke RB, Anderson E.
Oestrogens, Beatson and endocrine therapy.
Endocrine Rel Cancer 1997; **4**: 371–380.

4. Toniolo PG, Levitz M, Zeleniuch-Jacquotte A
et al. A prospective study of endogenous
estrogens and breast cancer in postmenopausal
women. *J Natl Cancer Inst* 1995; **87**:
190–197.

5. Lønning PE, Helle SI, Johannessen DC *et al.*
Influence of plasma oestrogen levels on the
length of the disease-free interval in
postmenopausal women with breast cancer.
Br Cancer Res Treat 1996; **39**: 335–341.

6. Berrino F, Muti P, Micheli A *et al.* Serum sex
hormone levels after menopause and
subsequent breast cancer. *J Natl Cancer Inst*
1996; **88**: 291–296.

7. Thomas HV, Key TJ, Allen DS *et al.* A
prospective study of endogenous serum
hormone concentrations and breast cancer
risk in post-menopausal women on the
island of Guernsey. *Br J Cancer* 1997; **76**:
401–405.

8. Hankinson SE, Willett WC, Manson JE *et al.*
Plasma sex steroid levels and risk of breast
cancer in postmenopausal women. *J Natl
Cancer Inst* 1998; **90**: 1292–1299.

9. Cauley JA, Lucas FL, Kuller LH *et al.*
Elevated serum estradiol and testosterone
concentrations are associated with a high risk
for breast cancer. *Ann Intern Med* 1999; **130**:
270–277.

10. Early Breast Cancer Trialists' Collaborative
Group. Ovarian ablation in early breast
cancer: overview of the randomised trials.
Lancet 1996; **348**: 1189–1196.

11. Early Breast Cancer Trialists' Collaborative
Group. Tamoxifen for early breast cancer: an
overview of randomised trials. *Lancet* 1998;
351: 1451–1467.

12. Hermon C, Beral V. Breast cancer mortality
rates are levelling off or beginning to decline
in many western countries: analysis of time
trends, age-cohort and age-period models of
breast cancer mortality in 20 countries. *Br J
Cancer* 1996; **73**: 955–960.

13. Fisher B, Costantino JP, Wickerham DL *et al.*
Tamoxifen for prevention of breast cancer:
report of the National Surgical Adjuvant
Breast and Bowel Project P-1 study. *J Natl
Cancer Inst* 1998; **90**: 1371–1388.

14. Jordan VC, Glusman JE, Eckert S *et al.* Raloxifene reduces incident primary breast cancer: integrated data from multi-centre, double-blind, placebo-controlled, randomised trials in postmenopausal women. *Br Cancer Res Treat* 1998; **50**: 277 (Abstract).

15. Thijssen JH, Blankenstein MA. Endogenous oestrogens and androgens in normal and malignant endometrial and mammary tissues. *Eur J Cancer Clin Oncol* 1989; **25**: 1953–1959.

16. Yasamura T, Akami T, Mitsou M *et al.* The effect of adjuvant therapy with or without tamoxifen on the endocrine function of patients with breast cancer. *Jpn J Surg* 1990; **20**: 369–375.

17. Carter AC, Sedransk N, Kelley RM *et al.* Diethylstilbestrol: recommended dosages for different categories of breast cancer patients. *JAMA* 1977; **237**: 2079–2085.

18. Palshof T, Cartensen B, Mouridsen HT, Dombernowsky P. Adjuvant endocrine therapy in pre- and postmenopausal women with operable breast cancer. *Rev Endocr Rel Cancer* 1985; **S17**: 43–50.

19. Sutton R, Buzdar AV, Hortobagyi GN. Pregnancy and offspring after adjuvant chemotherapy in breast cancer patients. *Cancer* 1990; **65**: 847–850.

20. von Scholtz E, Johansson H, Wilking N *et al.* Influence of prior and subsequent pregnancy on breast cancer prognosis. *J Clin Oncol* 1995; **13**: 430–434.

21. Schairer C, Byrne C, Keyl PM *et al.* Menopausal estrogen and estrogen–progestin replacement therapy and risk of breast cancer. *Cancer Causes & Control* 1994; **6**: 416–424.

22. Taubes G. Epidemiology faces its limits. *Science* 1995; **269**: 164–169.

23. Nachtigall MJ, Smilen SW, Nacthigall RD *et al.* Incidence of breast cancer in a 22-year study of women receiving estrogen–progestin replacement therapy. *Obstet Gynaecol*, 1992; **80**: 827–830.

24. Armstrong BK. Oestrogen therapy after the menopause: boon or bane? *Med J Aust* 1988; **148**: 213–214.

25. Dupont WD, Page DL. Menopausal estrogen replacement therapy and breast cancer. *Arch Int Med* 1991; **151**: 67–72.

26. Steinberg KK, Thacker SB, Smith JS *et al.* A meta-analysis of the effect of estrogen replacement therapy on the risk of breast cancer. *JAMA* 1991; **265**: 1985–1990.

27. Grady D, Ernster V. Invited commentary: does hormone replacement therapy cause breast cancer? *Am J Epidemiol* 1991; **134**: 1396–1400.

28. Sillero-Arenas M, Delgado-Rodriguez M, Rodigues-Canteras R *et al.* Menopausal hormone replacement therapy and breast cancer: a meta-analysis. *Obstet Gynaecol* 1992; **79**: 286–294.

29. Colditz GA, Egan KM, Stampfer MJ. Hormone replacement therapy and risk of breast cancer: results from epidemiological studies. *Am J Obs Gynaecol* 1993; **168**: 1473–1480.

30. Collaborative Group on Hormonal Factors for Breast Cancer. Breast cancer and hormone replacement therapy: collaborative reanalysis from 51 individual epidemiological studies. *Lancet* 1997; **350**: 1047–1060.

31. Osin P, Crook T, Powles TJ, Gusterson B. Hormone status of in situ cancer in BRCA1 and BRCA2 mutation carriers. *Lancet* 1998; **351**: 1487.

32. Rebbeck TR, Levin AM, Eisen A *et al.* Breast

cancer after bilateral prophylactic oophorectomy in BRCA1 mutation carriers. *J Natl Cancer Inst* 1999; **91**: 1475–1479.

33. Dupont WD, Page DL, Parl FF *et al.* Estrogen replacement therapy in women with a history of proliferative breast disease. *Cancer* 1999; **85**: 1277–1283.

34. Cowan LD, Gordis L, Tonascia JA *et al.* Breast cancer incidence in women with progesterone deficiency. *Am J Epidemiol* 1981; **114**: 209–217.

35. Sainsbury R. Timing of surgery and the ovarian cycle. *Endocrine Rel Cancer* 1997; **4**: 251–254.

36. Pike MC, Bernstein L, Spicer DV. Exogenous hormones and breast cancer. In: Niederhuber JE, ed. *Current Therapy in Oncology.* St Louis: CV Mosby, 1993, 292–303.

37. Maudelonde T, Lavaud P, Salazar G *et al.* Progestin treatment depresses oestrogen receptor but not cathepsin D levels in needle aspirates of benign breast disease. *Br Cancer Res Treat* 1991; **19**: 95–102.

38. Plu-Bureau G, Le MG, Sitruk-Ware R *et al.* Progestin use and decreased risk of breast cancer in a cohort study of premenopausal women with benign breast disease. *Br J Cancer* 1994; **70**: 270–277.

39. Clarke CL, Sutherland R. Progestin regulation of cellular proliferation. *Endocrine Reviews* 1990; **11**: 266–301.

40. Wren BG. Hormonal replacement therapy and breast cancer. *Eur J Menopause*, 1995; **2**: 13–21.

41. Colditz GA, Rosner B for the Nurses' Health Study Research Group. Use of estrogen plus progestin is associated with greater increase in breast cancer risk than estrogen alone. *Am J Epidemiol* 1998; **147** (suppl): 64S.

42. Persson I, Weiderpass E, Bergstrom R, Schairer C. Risks of breast cancer and endometrial cancer after estrogen and estrogen-progestin replacement therapy. *Cancer Causes Control* 1999; **10**: 253–260.

43. Magnusson C, Baron J, Correia N *et al.* Breast cancer risk following long-term oestrogen- and oestrogen–progestin-replacement therapy. *Int J Cancer* 1999; **81**: 339–344.

44. Schairer C, Lubin J, Troisi R *et al.* Menopausal estrogen and estrogen–progestin replacement therapy and breast cancer risk. *JAMA* 2000; **283**: 485–491.

45. Ross RK, Paganini-Hill A, Wan PC, Pike MC. Effect of hormone replacement therapy and breast cancer risk: estrogen versus estrogen plus progestin. *J Natl Cancer Inst* 2000; **92**: 328–332.

46. Greendale GA, Reboussin BA, Sie A *et al.* Effects of estrogen and estrogen–progestin on mammographic parenchymal density. *Ann Intern Med* 1999; **130**: 262–269.

47. Byrne C, Schairer C, Wolfe J *et al.* Mammographic features and breast cancer risk: effects with time, age and menopausal status. *J Natl Cancer Inst* 1995; **87**: 1622–1629.

48. Hofseth LJ, Raafat Am, Osuch JR *et al.* Hormone replacement therapy with estrogen or estrogen plus medroxyprogesterone acetate is associated with increased epithelial proliferation in the normal postmenopausal breast. *J Clin Endocrinol Metab* 1999; **84**: 4559–4565.

49. Kavanagh AM, Mitchell H, Giles GG. Hormone replacement therapy and accuracy of mammographic screening. *Lancet* 2000; **355**: 270–274.

50. Harvey JA, Pinkerton JV, Herman CR. Short-term cessation of hormone replacement

therapy and improvement of mammographic specificity. *J Natl Cancer Inst* 1997; **89**: 1623–1625.

51. BASO Breast Speciality Group. The British Association of Surgical Oncology Guidelines for surgeons in the management of symptomatic breast disease in the UK (1998 revision). *Eur J Surg Oncol* 1998; **24**: 464–476.

52. Dhodapkar MV, Ingle JN, Ahmann DL. Estrogen replacement therapy withdrawal and regression of metastatic breast cancer. *Cancer* 1995; 75: 43–46.

53. Harvey SC, DiPiro PJ, Meyer JE. Marked regression of a nonpalpable breast cancer after cessation of HRT. *Am J Radiol* 1996; **167**: 394–395.

54. DeFriend DJ, Howell A, Nicholson RI *et al.* Investigation of a pure new antioestrogen (ICI 182780) in women with primary breast cancer. *Cancer Res* 1994; **54**: 408–414.

55. Hargreaves DF, Knox F, Swindell R *et al.* Epithelial proliferation and hormone receptor status in the normal postmenopausal breast and the effects of hormone replacement therapy. *Br J Cancer* 1998; **78**: 945–949.

56. Foidart JM, Colin C, Denoo X *et al.* Estradiol and progesterone regulate the proliferation of human breast epithelial cells. *Fertil Steril* 1998; **69**: 963–969.

57. Grodstein F, Stampfer MJ, Colditz GA *et al.* Postmenopausal hormone therapy and mortality. *New Engl J Med* 1997; **336**: 1769–1775.

58. Gambrell DR. Proposal to decrease the risk and improve the prognosis in breast cancer. *Am J Obstet Gynaecol* 1984; **150**: 119–128.

59. Criqui MH, Suarez L, Barrett-Connor EL *et al.* Postmenopausal estrogen use and mortality. *Am J Epidemiolol* 1988; **128**: 606–614.

60. Berkqvist L, Adami HO, Persson I *et al.* Prognosis after breast cancer diagnosis in women exposed to oestrogen and oestrogen–progestogen replacement therapy. *Am J Epidemiolol* 1989; **130**: 221–228.

61. Hunt K, Vessey M, McPherson K. Mortality in a cohort of long-term users of hormone replacement therapy: an updated analysis. *Br J Obstet Gynaecol* 1990; **97**: 1080–1086.

62. Henderson BE, Paganini-Hill A, Ross RK. Decreased mortality in users of oestrogen replacement therapy. *Arch Int Med* 1991; **151**: 75–78.

63. Strickland DM, Gambrell RD, Butzin CA *et al.* The relationship between breast cancer survival and prior postmenopausal estrogen use. *Obstet Gynaecol* 1992; **80**: 400–404.

64. Folsom AR, Mink PJ, Sellers TA *et al.* Hormonal replacement therapy and morbidity and mortality in a prospective study of postmenopausal women. *Am J Pub Health* 1995; **85**: 1128–1132.

65. Persson I, Yuen J, Berqvist L *et al.* Cancer incidence and mortality in women receiving estrogen and estrogen–progestin replacement therapy—long-term follow-up of a Swedish cohort. *Int J Cancer* 1996; **67**: 327–332.

66. Willis DB, Calle EE, Miracle-McMahill HL *et al.* Estrogen replacement therapy and risk of fatal breast cancer in a prospective cohort of postmenopausal women in the United States. *Cancer Causes & Control* 1996; 7: 449–457.

67. Sellers TA, Mink PJ, Cerhan JR *et al.* The role of hormone replacement therapy in the risk for breast cancer and total mortality in women with a family history of breast cancer. *Ann Intern Med* 1997; **127**: 973–980.

68. Fowble B, Hanlon A, Patchefsky A *et al.* Postmenopausal hormone replacement therapy: effect on diagnosis and outcome in early-stage invasive breast cancer treated with conservative surgery and radiation. *J Clin Oncol* 1999; **17**: 1680–1688.

69. Jernström H, Frenander J, Fernö M *et al.* Hormone replacement therapy before breast cancer diagnosis significantly reduces the overall death rate compared with never-use among 984 breast cancer patients. *Br J Cancer* 1999; **80**: 1453–1458.

70. Schairer C, Gail M, Byrne C *et al.* Estrogen replacement therapy and breast cancer survival in a large screening study. *J Natl Cancer Inst* 1999; **91**: 264–270.

71. Gapstur SM, Morrow M, Sellers TA. Hormone replacement therapy and risk of breast cancer with a favourable histology. *JAMA* 1999; **281**: 2091–2097.

72. Carpenter JS, Andykowski MA, Cordova M *et al.* Hot flashes in postmenopausal women treated for breast carcinoma. *Cancer* 1998; **82**: 1682–1691.

73. Fallowfield LJ, Leaity SK, Howell A *et al.* Assessment of quality of life in women undergoing hormonal therapy for breast cancer: validation of an endocrine symptom subscale for the FACT-B. *Breast Cancer Res Treat* 1999; **55**: 189–199.

74. Ganz PA, Desmond K, Bekin TR *et al.* Predictors of sexual health in women after a breast cancer diagnosis. *J Clin Oncol* 1999; **17**: 2371–2380.

75. Couzi RJ, Helzlsouer KL, Fetting JB. Prevalence of menopausal symptoms among women with a history of breast cancer and attitudes toward estrogen replacement therapy. *J Clin Oncol* 1995; **13**: 2737–2744.

76. Day R, Ganz PA, Costantino JP *et al.* Health-related quality of life and tamoxifen in breast cancer prevention: a report from the National Surgical Adjuvant Breast and Bowel Project P-1 study. *J Clin Oncol* 1999; **17**: 2659–2669.

77. Chenoy R, Hussain S, Tayob V *et al.* Effect of oral gamolenic acid for evening primrose oil on menopausal flushing. *BMJ* 1992; **308**: 501–503.

78. Barton DL, Loprinzi CL, Quella SK *et al.* Prospective evaluation of vitamin E for hot flashes in breast cancer survivors. *J Clin Oncol* 1998; **16**: 495–500.

79. Goldberg RM, Loprinzi CL, O Fallon JR *et al.* Transdermal clonidine for ameliorating tamoxifen-induced hot flashes. *J Clin Oncol* 1994; **12**: 155–158.

80. Quella SK, Loprinzi CL, Barton D *et al.* Evaluation of soy phytoestrogens for treatment of hot flashes in breast cancer survivors: a North Central Cancer Treatment Group Trial. *J Clin Oncol* 1999; **18**: 1068–1074.

81. Loprinzi CL, Pisnansky TM, Fonseca R *et al.* Pilot evaluation of venlaflexine hydrochloride for the therapy of hot flashes in cancer survivors. *J Clin Oncol* 1998; **16**: 2377–2381.

82. Quella SK, Loprinzi CL, Sloan JA *et al.* Long term use of megestrol acetate by cancer survivors for the treatment of hot flushes. *Cancer* 1998; **82**: 1784–1788.

83. Milner M, Sinnott M, Gasparao D *et al.* Climacteric symptoms, gonadotrophins, sex steroids and binding proteins with conjugated equine estrogen–progestin and tibolone over two years. *Menopause* 1996; **4**: 208–213.

84. Pasqualini JR, Kloosterboer HJ, Chetrite G. Action of tibolone and its metabolites (org-

4094, Org-20126) on the biosynthesis and metabolism of estradiol in human breast cancer cells. *Breast Cancer Res Treat* 1998; **50**: P363 (Abstract).

85. Johannes E, Coelingh Bennick HJT, Engelen S *et al.* Tibolone: dose–response analysis of effects in climacteric symptoms. *Acta Obstet & Gynaecologica Scand* 1997; **76** (suppl 167): 5 FC801.6 (Abstract).

86. Stoll BA. Hormone replacement therapy in women treated for breast cancer. *Eur J Cancer Clin Oncol* 1989; **25**: 1909–1913.

87. Wile AG, Opfell RW, Margileth DA. Hormone replacement therapy in previously treated breast cancer patients. *Am J Surgery* 1993; **165**: 372–375.

88. DiSaia PJ, Odicino F, Grosen EA *et al.* Hormone replacement therapy in breast cancer. *Lancet* 1993; **342**: 1232.

89. Powles TP, Casey S, O'Brien M *et al.* Hormone replacement after breast cancer. *Lancet* 1993; **342**: 60–61.

90. Eden JA, Bush T, Nand S *et al.* A case-controlled study of combined continuous oestrogen–progestogen replacement therapy amongst women with a personal history of breast cancer. *Menopause* 1995; **2**; 67–72.

91. Vassilopoulou-Sellin R, Theriault R, Klein MJ. Estrogen replacement therapy in women with prior diagnosis and treatment for breast cancer. *Program/Proceedings of the 32nd Annual Meeting of the American Society of Clinical Oncology, Philadelphia, May 17–20 1996.* **15**: Abstract 50.

92. Peters GN, Jones SE. Estrogen replacement therapy in breast cancer patients: a time for change. *Program/Proceedings of the 32nd Annual Meeting of the American Society of Clinical Oncology, Philadelphia, May 17–20 1996.* **15**: Abstract 148.

93. Decker D, Cox T, Burdakin J *et al.* Hormone replacement therapy (HRT) in breast cancer survivors. *Program/Proceedings of the 32nd Annual Meeting of the American Society of Clinical Oncology, Philadelphia, May 17–20 1996.* **15**: Abstract 209.

94. Bluming AZ, Waisman JR, Dosik GM *et al.* Hormone replacement therapy in women with previously treated primary breast cancer. *Program/Proceedings of the 35th Annual Meeting of the American Society of Clinical Oncology, Atlanta, USA, May 17–19 1999.* **18**: Abstract 2285

95. Espie M, Gorins A, Perret F *et al.* Hormone replacement therapy (HRT) in patients treated for breast cancer: analysis of a cohort of 120 patients. *Program/Proceedings of the 35th Annual Meeting of the American Society of Clinical Oncology, Atlanta, USA, May 17–19 1999.* **18**: Abstract 2262.

96. Natrajan PK, Soumakis K, Gambrell D. Estrogen replacement therapy in women with previous breast cancer. *Am J Obstet Gynecol* 1999; **181**: 288–295.

97. Uršič-Vrščaj M, Bebar S. A case–control study of hormone replacement therapy after primary surgical breast cancer treatment. *Eur J Surg Oncol* 1999; **25**: 146–151.

98. Marsden J, Sacks, NPM, Baum M *et al.* Are randomised trials of hormone replacement therapy in symptomatic breast cancer patients feasible? *Fertility and Sterility* 2000; **73**: 292–299.

99. Powles TJ, Eeles R, Ashley S *et al.* Interim analysis of breast cancer in the Royal Marsden Hospital tamoxifen randomised chemoprevention trial. *Lancet* 1998; **352**: 98–101.

100. Veronesi U, Maisonneuve P, Costa A *et al.*

Prevention of breast cancer with tamoxifen: preliminary findings from the Italian randomised trial among hysterectomised women. *Lancet* 1998; **352**: 93–97.

101. Chang J, Powles TJ, Ashley SE *et al.* The effect of tamoxifen and hormone replacement therapy on serum cholesterol, bone mineral density and coagulation factors in healthy postmenopausal women participating in a randomised, controlled tamoxifen prevention study. *Ann Oncol* 1996; **7**: 671–675.

102. Chang J, Powles TJ, Ashley SE *et al.* Variation in endometrial thickening in women with amenorrhoea. *Br Cancer Res Treat* 1998; **48**: 81–85.

103. Ederveen AGH, Kloosterboer HJ. Tibolone, a tissue selective steroid, exerts its preventive action on trabecular bone loss in ovariectomised rats through the estrogen receptor. *J Bone Min Res* 1996; **11** (suppl): 349 (Abstract).

104. Decensi A, Robertson C, Rotmensz N *et al.* Effect of tamoxifen and transdermal hormone replacement therapy on cardiovascular risk factors in a prevention trial. *Br J Cancer* 1998; **78**: 572–578.

105. Cauley J, Krueger K, Eckert S *et al.* Raloxifene reduces breast cancer risk in postmenopausal women with osteoporosis: 40-month data from the MORE trial. *Program/Proceedings of the 35th Annual Meeting of the American Society of Clinical Oncology, Atlanta, USA, May 17–19 1999.* **18**: Abstract 328.

Selective oestrogen receptor modulators

David W Purdie, Clare E Kearney

12

Introduction

Precision in targeting is, in general, as desirable an objective in the field of pharmacology as it is on the field of battle. Adverse clinical effects, known elsewhere as collateral damage, often result from the inadvertent or indeed unavoidable engagement of sites whose structural similarity or proximity to the true target places them literally in the firing line. Hence, several of the 20th century's great advances in therapeutics, such as cardioselective β blockade, selective H_2 antagonism, and, most recently, specific COX-2 inhibition, have closely followed sharper identification of the target structure. Indeed, a central goal of biochemistry is the delineation of isoforms, those variable molecular species of a generic molecule such as a receptor, with the aim not only of elucidating structure and function but also of securing precision in stimulation or inhibition as clinical need may demand.

In the case of oestrogens, the first half century of their therapeutic use may be seen in retrospect as the era of the blunderbuss rather than the bullet. The utilization of human oestradiol-17β or conjugated equine oestrogens provided many benefits to patients but also brought adverse effects principally due to the actions of these oestrogens upon two of their principal target tissues—the breast and the uterus. Hence the development of selective oestrogen receptor modulators (SERMs) may be seen conceptually as an attempt to delete the reproductive system from the array of oestrogen response tissues while maintaining activity in those non-reproductive systems where oestrogen action contributes to normal function. The evolution of the SERMs is therefore set to follow an algorithmic path that will specify progressive refinement in their design as we seek to include within their therapeutic range all those physiological systems upon which evolution has bestowed a role for oestrogen. Given that we remain ignorant of the full range of oestrogen actions, especially those mediated by cell membrane receptors and second messengers rather than by gene transcription, this field will remain one of intense scientific activity for the foreseeable future.

Evolution

If one accepts Gordhansky's famous phrase 'Nothing in biology makes sense except in terms of evolution', then the group of steroid hormones known as the oestrogens have indeed conferred survival advantage through their involvement in many vertebrate physiological systems. The simplest living organism that has been shown to possess an oestrogen receptor and oestradiol 17β as ligand is the eukaryotic unicellular yeast *Saccharomyces cerevisiae.*[1] Among multicellular animals the oestrogens are found first in the phylum Echinodermata, represented today by the starfish, and in the phylum Mollusca, represented by the octopus and squid, whose ancestors, evolving from simpler forms some 400 million years ago, were apparently the first to possess the cytochrome P450 aromatase enzyme system necessary to convert C-19 androgens to C-18 oestrogens.[2] Studies of steroid hormone evolution show that in comparison the glucocorticoids and mineralocorticoids are of more recent origin, appearing first in the elasmobranchs—sharks and rays—and that aldosterone is first found in the teleosts or bony fish. When one considers that it was only 6 million years ago that the evolutionary line leading to *Homo sapiens* branched away from the line leading to our nearest cousin, *Pan troglodytes*, the chimpanzee, it can be seen that our species inherited a signalling system that had been part of physiology for the major part of eukaryotic life on earth. Nature is parsimonious. A molecule that possesses a set of physico-chemical characteristics that are of advantage in a primitive system may be retained to discharge its function in more complex evolving systems provided that such new functions do not confer a net disadvantage upon survival.

The oestrogens' primal and still central

role is in reproduction. Darwinian theory requires that no significant compromise of reproductive efficiency will be tolerated; this is attested by the observation that the pattern of oestradiol seen in adult human plasma is that imposed by the reproductive cycle.

The mid-cycle peak of plasma oestradiol synthesized in the granulosa cells of growing follicles stimulates the luteinizing hormone (LH) surge from the anterior pituitary, which in turn triggers the eruption of the mature ovum on to the ovarian surface. A secondary plasma surge of oestradiol is produced by the corpus luteum in the secretory phase of the cycle. Overall, the oestradiol plasma values are those that oestrogen replacement therapy seeks to reproduce (see *Fig. 12.1*).

Without exception, all the non-reproductive activities of oestrogens must accommodate to this unvarying plasma pattern, just as they must accommodate to the plasma levels of oestrogen which pertain during pregnancy and lactation. In the evolutionary context it should be noted that, in the absence of contraception, hominid and, later, human females would experience relatively few menstrual cycles given the intense reproductive activity that separated puberty and death.

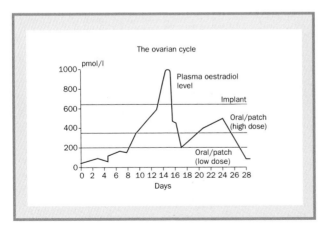

Figure 12.1
Plasma oestradiol over a 28 day cycle, showing levels achievable by replacement regimens.

Oestrogen receptor: structure and function

The oestrogen receptor belongs to the steroid receptor superfamily, which comprises the glucocorticoid, vitamin D, thyroid hormone, androgen, and retinoid receptors—whose modular construction with its highly conserved DNA-binding domains bespeaks a common evolutionary origin for these complex proteins.[3] (See *Fig. 12.2*.)

The receptors reside in the nucleus, cloaked by heatshock proteins (HSP) until the arrival of ligand. Physiologically, ligand is usually oestradiol or oestrone which is incorporated into the large binding cavity of the oestrogen receptor (ER), thereby triggering conformational change as the activated receptor dimerizes, casts off the HSP, and displays binding sites for a range of co-activators and co-repressors that modulate its subsequent activity.[4] (See *Fig. 12.3*.)

The oestrogen–ER complex now seeks the palindromic promotor sequences of oestrogen response elements in target genes. The complex then proceeds to facilitate RNA transcriptase and messenger RNA. An essential feature of ER action is the differential activity of the transcriptase activation areas AF-1 and AF-2.[5]

AF-1 is thought to be constitutive, that is, it operates without the presence of ligand, whereas AF-2 requires the presence of oestradiol or a substitute in the binding cavity of the receptor.

First generation

Compounds known as first-generation SERMs were originally classed as anti-oestrogens until it was found that their actions were more complex and contained an admixture of agonist and antagonist activities.

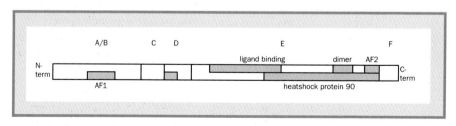

Figure 12.2
Schematic representation of the oestrogen receptor with six domains (A–F).

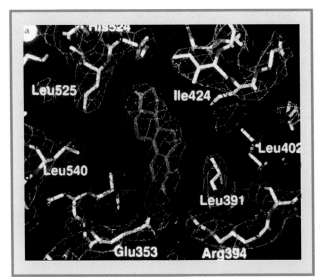

Figure 12.3
Electron crystallographic map of the ER-binding pocket with oestradiol in situ. Reproduced from reference 4, with permission.

Clomiphene citrate, a triphenylethylene, was synthesized in 1956 and was found by Greenblatt *et al* in 1961 to be capable of inducing ovulation in infertile women,[6] a clinical role that it performs to this day. The central action of clomiphene is to block the negative feedback of oestrogen and to induce, through positive feedback, a follicle stimulating hormone (FSH) surge from the gonadotrophs of the anterior pituitary. In 1984 it was observed that clomiphene attenuated bone loss in the oophorectomized (OVX) rat.[7] This was most surprising, since, intuitively, an anti-oestrogen with some

oestrogenic activity would have been expected to promote rather than retard bone loss in this animal model. However, clomiphene is not a pure chemical entity but a combination of two geometric isomers. The *trans* isomer enclomiphene is a partial oestrogen whereas the *cis* isomer zuclomiphene is a pure oestrogen. The molecular species responsible for clomiphene's remarkable effect on rat bone could thus not be ascertained.

Subsequently, another triphenylethylene, tamoxifen, was similarly shown to prevent bone loss in the OVX rat and it later became clear that this agent, now in general use as adjunctive therapy in breast cancer, was also operating as an oestrogen agonist in the skeleton and the cardiovascular system.[8,9] Clomiphene and tamoxifen were thus exposed as selective oestrogens and it was immediately apparent that such compounds could be of great potential benefit in supplying oestrogenic action in such tissues as bone, heart, and brain while antagonizing oestrogenic action in breast and uterus. Tamoxifen was not further developed as a bone-sparing agent, however, due to concerns over its propensity to cause uterine stimulation in some women. This has amounted to endometrial hyperplasia and adenocarcinoma in some reported cases.[10]

Second generation: raloxifene

Raloxifene, originally styled keoxifene, emerged from the Eli Lilly research laboratories in the USA as one of an array of benzothiophenes synthesized for potential use in the treatment of breast cancer.[11] Raloxifene is not a steroid and hence not technically an oestrogen but it possesses the vital phenolic ring—similar to the A ring of oestradiol— necessary to obtain lodgement in the ligand-binding cavity of the ER (see *Fig. 12.4*).

In the normal course of events, natural ligand binding is followed by dimerization and the phosphorylation of certain serine and threonine residues.[12] The reconfigured ER binding now presents active surfaces for the attachment of co-activators or co-repressors.[13] With raloxifene in situ, however, a key difference emerges in receptor activity. Unlike oestradiol, the molecule has an alkylaminoethoxy side chain, which physically and functionally protrudes from the binding domain and binds to an aminoacid residue (aspartate) at position 351 in the ER

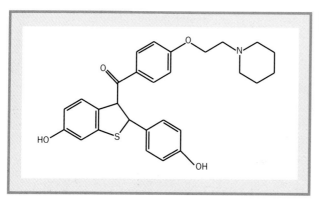

Figure 12.4
Structure of raloxifene.

structure.[14] This has a splinting effect and prevents the rotation of helix 12 of the ER, which has the dual action of closing up the occupied binding domain and permitting the AF-2 domain of the ER to proceed to normal activation of RNA transcriptase II.[15] (See *Fig. 12.5*.) With raloxifene as ligand, the splinted helix 12 cannot undergo the rotation, with the result that the AF-2 function is disabled.[4] Raloxifene thus acts as an AF-2 inhibitor, and in tissues such as the breast and uterus where an operational AF-2 is required for oestrogen action, no oestrogenic action occurs. The key role of aspartate 351 in the action of raloxifene was elegantly demonstrated by Levenson and Jordan,[14] who showed that a natural mutation of aspartate to tyrosine at this position reversed raloxifene's oestrogen antagonism to agonism in human breast cancer cells.

Raloxifene: clinical actions

Bone

The central pathophysiological process in postmenopausal bone loss is accelerated turnover of bone and an associated imbalance

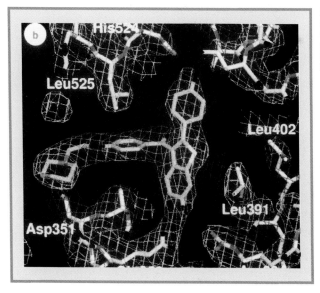

Figure 12.5
Electron crystallographic map of the ER-binding pocket, with raloxifene in situ. Reproduced from reference 4, with permission.

between bone formation and resorption in favour of the latter. (See *Fig. 12.6.*)

Thus, the desired end-points of oestrogen or SERM action in bone are a restraint on turnover, measured by a decline in plasma or urine turnover markers and a stabilization, or indeed a gain, in bone mineral density (BMD). An observed decline in clinical fracture at the key sites of vertebrae, distal radius, and femoral neck is the desired clinical outcome.

Using the isotope ^{45}Ca, Heaney and Draper found that raloxifene in a dose of 60 mg/day significantly reduced urinary calcium excretion without significant change in calcium absorption from the gut.[16] These data were interpreted as indicating a significant fall in calcium of bone origin being presented to the kidneys. In other words, bone resorption had been impeded. No change in bone formation by raloxifene was found. Support for the notion that raloxifene reduced bone resorption came from the work of Draper *et al*, who reported an 8 week study of healthy postmenopausal women.[17] These

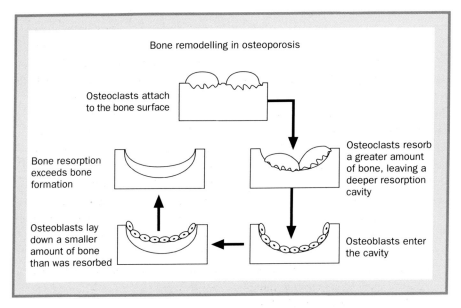

Figure 12.6
The bone turnover cycle in conditions of oestrogen deficiency.

workers found that raloxifene induced a significant reduction in serum bone-specific alkaline phosphatase and osteocalcin, which represent bone formation, and in urinary hydroxyproline and pyridinoline crosslinks, which represent bone resorption. This suggestion of a raloxifene-induced slowdown in turnover was supported by Delmas *et al* in a larger and randomized, placebo-controlled study of 601 postmenopausal non-osteoporotic women.[18] Raloxifene, in a dose of 60 mg/day, induced a significant fall in serum alkaline phosphatase, osteocalcin, and also urinary type I collagen C-telopeptide, the latter reflecting bone resorption, over a 24 month period. The translation of reduced turnover into maintenance of BMD was also examined in the study and it was shown that raloxifene-treated patients exhibited at 24 months a percentage BMD gain of 2.4 ± 0.4 at the spine and of 2.4 ± 0.4 at the hip. That these gains were not being achieved at the expense of bone mineral density elsewhere was attested by a total body bone mineral density gain of 2.0 ± 0.4 ($p < 0.001$). In the above study all participants were rendered calcium replete by supplementation with a minimum of 400 mg of elemental calcium daily and hence the effects on bone are indeed likely to be caused by raloxifene.

Data on raloxifene and vertebral fracture have recently appeared in a report by Ettinger *et al* on 3 years' experience with raloxifene in the MORE (Multiple Outcomes of Raloxifene Evaluation) study, which enrolled 7705 osteoporotic women, randomized to receive placebo, raloxifene 60 mg/day, or raloxifene 120 mg/day.[19] All participants received calcium / vitamin D supplements. Bone density measurement was by dual energy X-ray absorptiometry (DEXA) at 12 month intervals and vertebral deformation and fracture were assessed blindly on a semiquantitative scale of 0–3 as described by Genant *et al.*[20] Overall, the relative risk of a first vertebral fracture in a raloxifene-treated patient receiving 60 mg/day was 0.70 (95% CI, 0.50–0.80). Protection was present whether or not patients had a pre-existing vertebral fracture. When such a fracture was present the risk of a subsequent fracture was 0.70 (95% CI, 0.60–0.90); when it was not, the risk fell to 0.5 (95% CI, 0.40–0.80). The 60 mg/day raloxifene regimen increased BMD at the femoral neck by 2.1%, which was significantly greater than in the controls ($p < 0.001$) but neither at this nor at any other non-spine site was any difference in fracture incidence found (RR 0.9; 95% CI, 0.8–1.1). The vertebral fracture protection data are encouraging but it remains to be seen whether the all-important long-term effect of femoral neck fracture prevention will be achieved. Further interventive studies on older populations will be required to rest such a proposal.

Cardiovascular system

A wealth of observational data support the concept of oestrogens being active in the primary prevention of atherosclerosis and subsequent cardiovascular events (see Chapters 5, 6, 7 and 8). It would obviously be desirable if such activity extended to SERMs, and this has been a major area of study. It is important to stress that all studies to date have examined cardiovascular disease from the viewpoint of primary prevention. The role of oestrogen as a secondary preventive agent in patients with existing disease is contentious—following the publication of the Heart and Estrogen/progestin Replacement Study (HERS) in 1998, in which there was an excess of cardiovascular events in the hormone replacement therapy (HRT) group compared with controls during the first 12 months of study.[21] An examination of the effect of raloxifene on lipid profile behaviour was reported by Walsh et al.[22] In this randomized, placebo-controlled trial, the standard dose of 60 mg/day raloxifene induced significant falls of some 12% in low density lipoprotein cholesterol (LDL-C) and of 8% in lipoprotein(a). Although no change was found in the level of the protective high density lipoprotein cholesterol (HDL-C) there was a significant rise in the HDL_2-C subfraction. No change was found in the level of triglycerides or in plasminogen activator inhibitor 1. On the blood coagulation front,

raloxifene lowered plasma fibrinogen significantly and did not change fibrinopeptide A or either of the prothrombin fragments. In the study of Delmas et al the 60 mg daily raloxifene regimen, given to some 152 women over 2 years produced a similar picture with a significant reduction in LDL-C and no change in HDL-C and triglycerides.[18] This group did not report on indices of blood coagulation or fibrinolysis.

Thus, the picture is complex and significantly different from that wrought by conventional oral HRT therapy with its significant fall in total circulating cholesterol and rise in triglycerides. In animal studies a confused picture has emerged. Raloxifene inhibits the accumulation of cholesterol in the aorta of oophorectomized rabbits[23] whereas in a primate model Clarkson et al failed to detect any effect of raloxifene on coronary artery atherogenesis in cynomolgus monkeys.[24] No human studies have yet been powered to detect changes in clinical cardiovascular endpoints and hence no statement can yet be made as to whether the above-mentioned lipid change will translate into clinical effect. In MORE, all-cause mortality over 3 years did not differ between the raloxifene-treated and the control groups.

Effects on the breast

In many studies one of the prime disincentives to the acceptance or continuation of conventional HRT is the perceived risk of breast cancer,[25] which remains the most common malignancy in UK females. Since raloxifene was originally synthesized as one of a group of benzothiphenes for potential use in breast cancer, it has been of considerable interest to examine its effect on this malignancy in controlled trials.

Recently Cummings *et al*[26] reported that among the 5129 women in the MORE trial randomized to receive raloxifene there developed, over the subsequent 3 years, 13 cases of invasive breast cancer. Among the 2576 placebo-treated controls there developed 27 cases of invasive breast cancer. The overall relative risk of breast cancer in treated women was 0.24 (95% CI, 0.13–0.44). As with tamoxifen, the effect appears to be concentrated against the more common ER-positive cancers, the relative risk of which, again compared with placebo, fell to a remarkable 0.10 (95% CI, 0.04–0.24). In contrast, ER-negative cancers showed no change (RR = 0.88, 95% CI, 0.26–3.0). However, numbers of these latter tumours were small, as evidenced by the wide confidence interval. Since mammograms of treated patients do not show the increase in radio-opacity found with HRT regimens, it is unlikely that any observational or test bias was operating. It should be understood that breast cancer prevention was a secondary not a primary end-point of MORE, and the study population, being osteoporotic, were at no

excess risk of the disease. However, the incidence of invasive breast cancer in the control group was no different than that expected for this population and it would appear, prima facie, that a useful effect is present. Given that breast tumours are present for months or even years before coming to clinical notice it is likely that the raloxifene effect is one of suppression rather than primary prevention. Hence, it will be necessary to follow up a significant number of patients exiting the study to detect any rebound phenomenon. The ability of raloxifene to reduce the incidence of invasive breast cancer in a group of women at high risk is being explored in the Study of Tamoxifen and Raloxifene (STAR) now recruiting in North America.

Adverse effects of treatment

Raloxifene is generally well tolerated. In the MORE study less than one in 10 of participants withdrew due to an adverse event, although it should be noted that in the study of Delmas *et al* the dropout rate was 25%, the reasons for which were unspecified by the authors.[18] Experience in the MORE study was that side-effects were usually mild and transient, the most common being vasomotor symptoms, hot flushes and sweats, calf cramps, and peripheral oedema.[19] More significant was the incidence of venous thromboembolic phenomena. In MORE there were 18 DVTs and 10 pulmonary emboli among the group receiving 60 mg daily raloxifene, the numbers among the placebo group being five and three, respectively. Overall, the relative risk of venous thrombo-embolism (VTE) in the raloxifene group compared with placebo was 3.1 (95% CI, 1.5–6.2),[26] an increase comparable to that consistently found with conventional HRT.[27,28] Given that raloxifene reduces plasma fibrinogen and does not appear to inhibit fibrinolysis, no explanation for these data is presently available and is urgently required.

Effects on the uterus

The uterus is of course exquisitively sensitive to oestrogen, responding to oestradiol stimulation with increased blood flow and endometrial proliferation. Given that the avoidance of cyclic or unscheduled bleeding is a prime objective in terms of adherence to oestrogen therapy, the uterine effects of raloxifene have been carefully studied. Clinically, patients receiving 60 mg raloxifene in the MORE study reported a 3.4% incidence of vaginal bleeding, no different from the rate occurring among placebo-treated controls.[26] At 40 months of follow-up, there had been only 10 cases of endometrial cancer among the total enrollment of 7705. The relative risk of this tumour among raloxifene-treated women was 0.8 (95% CI, 0.2–2.7). The absence of bleeding is a most welcome

clinical development as is the apparent lack of effect on uterine cancer, given that cyclic HRT regimens may be associated with such tumours.

Conclusion

The first of the second-generation SERMs was licensed in 1998. During that time two other agents, levormeloxifene and idoxifene, have been withdrawn from clinical trial because of adverse events, principally endometrial stimulation and, in the case of idoxifene, an excess of cases of uterovaginal prolapse. Raloxifene, however, appears to be well tolerated and the general absence of breast and uterine adverse events is a significant advantage. Patients do not, however, achieve a reduction in menopausal symptoms, and where such are a clinical problem conventional HRT must retain the central role. Similarly, there are as yet no data on the ability of raloxifene to control the vaginal dryness and associated dyspareunia that can be so distressing to postmenopausal women; here again systemic or local oestrogen therapy is indicated. Future studies with SERMs will need to address the issue of cardiovascular protection, cognitive function, and neurodegeneration.

The patient in whom the use of a SERM is indicated is a postmenopausal women at risk of osteoporosis-related vertebral fracture. These agents will be of particular value in patients who have experienced adverse events during HRT therapy or who are unable to accept bleeding or the small but quantifiable increased risk of breast cancer. For the present, in a patient at risk of osteoporosis, a general schedule for oestrogen use after menopause might involve the use of conventional HRT for the vital sixth decade—the decade after menopause—followed by an actuarial assessment of future fracture risk using validated clinical risk factors and BMD measurement by DEXA of the hip and spine. In patients manifesting significant risk of fracture—the risk roughly doubles for each standard deviation fall in BMD—the option will be to switch to an SERM or to continue with conventional HRT or use a bisphosphonate. Densitometric follow-up will be required and all women at risk should make any necessary lifestyle adjustment to take a diet that is calcium / vitamin D replete and an activity pattern producing adequate weight-bearing exercise.

The SERMs are a major step forward in therapeutics. They are the fruit of our new understanding of the complexity of oestrogen receptor structure and function, a complexity that has been correctly seen not as an obstacle but as an opportunity. These purpose-designed agents will, with increasing sophistication, maintain oestrogenic action wherever in physiology the hormone and its receptor have been adopted as a signal transduction system, while dispensing with those reproductive actions that become redundant with menopause and whose reactivation is, at best, an encumbrance and, at worst, a clinical hazard.

References

1. Feldman D, Tökés LG, Stathis PA *et al.* Identification of 17β-estradiol as the estrogenic substance in *Saccharomyces cerevisiae. Proc Natl Acad Sci* 1984; **81**: 4722–4726.

2. Sandor T, Mehdi AZ. Steroids and evolution. In: Barrington EJW, ed. *Hormones and Evolution.* New York: Academic Press, 1979, 1–72.

3. Laudet V, Hänni C, Coll J *et al.* Evolution of the nuclear receptor gene family. *EMBO J* 1992; **11**: 1003–1013.

4. Brzozowski AM, Pike ACW, Dauter Z *et al.* Molecular basis of agonism and antagonism in the oestrogen receptor. *Nature* 1997; **389**: 753–758.

5. Ekena K, Weis KE, Katzenellenbogen JA *et al.* Different residues of the human estrogen receptor are involved in the recognition of structurally diverse estrogens and antiestrogens. *J Biol Chem* 1997; **272**: 5069–5075.

6. Greenblatt RB, Barfield WE, Jungck EC *et al.* Induction of ovulation with MRI-41. *JAMA* 1961; **178**: 101–106.

7. Beall PT, Misra KL, Young RL, Spjut HJ *et al.* Clomiphene protects against osteoporosis in the mature ovariectomized rat. *Calcif Tissue Int* 1985; **36**: 123–135.

8. Jordan VC, Phelps E, Lindgren JU. Effects of anti-estrogens on bone in castrated and intact female rats. *Breast Can Res Treat* 1987; **10**: 31–35.

9. Love RR, Barden HS, Mazess RB *et al.* Effect

of tamoxifen on lumbar spine bone mineral density in postmenopausal women after 5 years. *Arch Intern Med* 1994; **154**: 2585–2588.

10. Ismail SM. Effect of tamoxifen on the uterus. *Lancet* 1994; **344**: 622–623.

11. Draper MW, Flowers DE, Neild JA *et al*. Antiestrogenic properties of raloxifene. *Pharmacology* 1995; **50**: 209–217.

12. Katzenellenbogen JA, O'Malley BW, Katzenellenbogen BS. Tripartite steroid hormone receptor pharmacology: interaction with multiple effector sites as a basis for the cell- and promoter-specific action of these hormones. *Mol Endocrinol* 1996; **10**: 119–131.

13. Beato M, Sanchez-Pácheco A. Interaction of steroid hormone receptors with the transcription initiation complex. *Endocr Rev* 1996; **17**: 587–609.

14. Levenson AS, Jordan VC. The key to the antiestrogenic mechanism of raloxifene is amino acid 351 (aspartate) in the estrogen receptor. *Can Res* 1998; **58**: 1872–1875.

15. Tsai MJ, O'Malley BW. Molecular mechanisms of action of steroid/thyroid receptor superfamily members. *Ann Rev Biochem* 1994; **63**: 451–486.

16. Heaney RP, Draper MW. Raloxifene and estrogen: comparative bone-remodeling kinetics. *J Clin Endocrinol Metab* 1997; **82**: 3425–3429.

17. Draper MW, Flowers DE, Huster WJ *et al*. A controlled trial of raloxifene (LY139481) HCl: impact on bone turnover and serum lipid profile in healthy postmenopausal women. *J Bone Min Res* 1996; **11**: 835–842.

18. Delmas PD, Bjarnason NH, Mitlak BH *et al*. Effects of raloxifene on bone mineral

density, serum cholesterol concentrations and uterine endometrium in postmenopausal women. *New Engl J Med* 1997; **337**: 1641–1647.

19. Ettinger B, Black DM, Mitlak BH *et al*. Reduction of vertebral fracture risk in postmenopausal women with osteoporosis treated with raloxifene. *JAMA* 1999; **282**: 637–645.

20. Genant HK, Jergas M, Palermo *et al* for the Study of Osteoporotic Fractures Research Group. Comparison of semiquantitative visual and quantitative morphometric assessment of prevalent and incident vertebral fractures in osteoporosis. *J Bone Miner Res* 1996; **11**: 984–996.

21. Hulley S, Grady D, Bush T *et al*. Randomized trial of estrogen plus progestin for secondary prevention of coronary heart disease in postmenopausal women. *JAMA* 1998; **280**: 605–613.

22. Walsh BW, Kuller LH, Wild RA *et al*. Effects of raloxifene on serum lipids and coagulation factors in healthy postmenopausal women. *JAMA* 1998; **279**: 1445–1451.

23. Bjarnason NH, Haarbo J, Byrjalsen I *et al*. Raloxifene inhibits aortic accumulation of cholesterol in ovariectomized, cholesterol-fed rabbits. *Circulation* 1997; **96**: 1964–1969.

24. Clarkson TB, Anthony MS, Jerome CP. Lack of effect of raloxifene on coronary artery atherosclerosis of postmenopausal monkeys. *J Clin Endocrinol Metab* 1998; **83**: 721–726.

25. Purdie DW, Steel SA, Howey S, Doherty SM. The technical and logistical feasibility of population densitometry using DXA and directed HRT intervention: a 2-year prospective study. *Osteoporos Int* 1996; **6**(suppl 3): 31–36.

26. Cummings SR, Eckert S, Krueger KA *et al*.

The effect of raloxifene on risk of breast cancer in postmenopausal women. Results from the MORE randomized trial. *JAMA* 1999; **281**: 2189–2197.

27. Jick H, Derby LE, Myers MW *et al.* Risk of hospital admission for idiopathic venous thromboembolism among users of postmenopausal oestrogens. *Lancet* 1996; **348**: 981–983.

28. Daly E, Vessey MP, Hawkins MM *et al.* Risk of venous thromboembolism in users of hormone replacement therapy. *Lancet* 1996; **348**: 977–980.

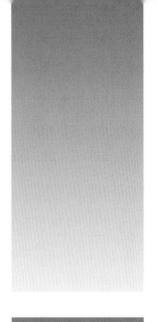

Index

Numbers in italics indicate *tables* and *figures*.

route of administration-related 8
see also abnormal vaginal bleeding
small dense LDLs 74, 103
sociocultural factors and the menopause 15
soy phyto-oestrogens 143
statins 72, 80
steroid hormone evolution 158–9
St John's wort 5
stress and abnormal bleeding 5
stress incontinence
    oestrogen treatment 33–4, 37
    prevalence 31, *32*
stress management 22
stroke and HRT 66, 117–19, *118*
Study of Tamoxifen and Raloxifene (STAR)
    167
surveillance bias 142

tachyphylaxis 8
tamoxifen
    clinical effects 147
    and HRT 5, 146–8
    hyperoestrogenic state induction 134
    as a selective oestrogen 161–2
testosterone
    addition to oestrogen 9, 51
    implants 9
TGFβ *see* transforming growth factor β
thrombophilia screens 2
tibolone 50
    in diabetics 110
    and HDL levels 79
    and lipoprotein(a) levels 77
    prevention of LDL oxidation 76

and triglyceride levels 77, 78
vascular effects 96
TNFα (tumour necrosis factor α) 44, *45*
topical oestrogen 143
transforming growth factor β (TGFβ) 44, 45,
    45, 76
transient ischaemic attacks 115, 119
transvaginal ultrasound 6
travel and abnormal bleeding 5
triglyceride-rich lipoproteins
    and HRT 77–8, 91
    and insulin resistance 103
tumour necrosis factor α (TNFα) 44, *45*
Turner's syndrome 128–9
urethra, effects of oestrogen 28–9
urge incontinence
    causes *34*
    oestrogen treatment 34–5, 37
    prevalence 31, *32*
urinary incontinence *see* stress incontinence;
    urge incontinence
urinary sediment 29
urinary symptoms
    effects of progesterone 29–30
    oestrogen treatment *31*, 32
    relation to menstrual cycle 29, *30*
    see also stress incontinence; urge
        incontinence
urinary tract infections 35
    oestrogen treatment 35–7, *36*

Vabra curettes 7
vaginal bleeding
    abnormal *see* abnormal vaginal bleeding